Perioperative Pearls for the Novice

A Primer for the Health Care Student

Carl F. Giesler, MD and Harold J. Miller, MD

To order additional copies of this book, contact:
Xlibris
844-714-8691
www.Xlibris.com
Orders@Xlibris.com

ISBN: Softcover   978-1-6641-7850-2
       Hardcover   978-1-6641-7851-9
       EBook   978-1-6641-7849-6

Library of Congress Control Number: 2021911356

Print information available on the last page

Rev. date: 06/17/2022

To our wives, Kathy Giesler and Rici Miller for allowing us to spend so much time away from them while working on this project. They understand our years of commitment to education and the importance of sharing our knowledge with tomorrow's health-care providers in this primer.

Contents

Preface

Why did we decide to publish another book on basic surgical concepts in 2021?

Surgical skills and theories have increased geometrically since the 1940s. Surgical training was initially taught by the mentor-apprentice tradition. Now it is taught in groups and simulation labs using virtual reality. Along the evolution pathway, some of the basic reasons for doing things in a certain way have been lost.

The surgical literature is full of articles and books that describe multiple pathways to perform and treat the same surgical condition. The authors have more than 110 years of combined surgical experience and want to share their experience, emphasizing certain basic principles that improve their surgical efficiency. This primer is a resource for the medical student, early resident surgeon, paramedical personnel, and practitioners enhancing their surgical knowledge and patient-care skills.

The authors do not presume that the techniques described in this primer are the only way to manage surgical issues. Many surgeons have solved similar issues using approaches different than those described in this primer. However, the techniques described in this primer have stood the test of time in the practices of Drs. Giesler and Miller. The authors also indicate areas of risk and discuss reasons for the risk. Using techniques described in this primer, the reader will learn safe approaches for management of many surgical issues and will minimize adverse outcomes for their patients.

Our pictures are more important than our words!

This primer has numerous illustrations. The importance of each illustration is discussed in the text adjacent to the figure. To use this primer most effectively, look at the illustration first, then read the associated text, and then, review the figure again.

This primer provides novice health-care students information to formulate sound patient-care decisions. Many situations presented in this primer illustrate non-surgical risks that affect patient outcome. The authors have written this primer to stimulate observation of the non-surgical obstacles that impact patient surgical outcomes.

Patient Safety in the OR

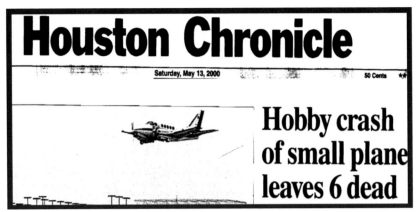

Ref 1

Federal investigators determined a removeable steel pin caused the crash that left six dead. The gust-lock pin prevents strong winds from moving a parked airplane's ailerons and elevators. The bent pin was found still in place in the control column in the plane wreckage. With the pin in place the pilot would have had no control over the plane in flight. Removing the pin is a basic step in a pilot's preflight routine as well as installing the pin is a normal post-flight procedure.

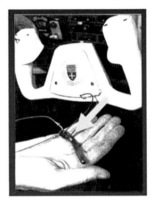

Ref 2

Details make the difference when providing patient safety in the OR.

This book is about those details.

Just as the pilot makes his pre-flight check of the airplane to confirm the plane is ready for a successful flight, the surgeon should confirm that their patient and the operating room (OR)are ready for their surgery. Patient safety in the OR begins prior to the patient ever entering the OR.

The authors have extensive surgical experience caring for patients in the OR. Much of their decision-making resulted from job experience and extensive self-assessment of their decision-making and outcomes of those decisions. Reasons for results were discussed with colleagues and literature review as well as personal analysis. Actions were changed as a result and influenced future decision-making in a positive way. Both authors have reviewed numerous malpractice cases as experts for both plaintiff and defendant attorneys during their professional career. This experience provided additional exposure to other instances of patient risk in the OR. The information that follows is an illustrated primer on risks patients have during a surgical procedure.

Patient Safety in the OR Begins as Part of the Preoperative Assessment

Technology continues to improve surgical management and patient outcomes for many conditions. Despite these medical advances, patients continue to experience pressure-induced injuries related to surgical positioning. These injuries happen because the anesthetized patient is unable to alert the surgeon of painful positions. Some patients are more at risk for surgical position problems than others. Identification of these patients during their preoperative visit allows the surgeon to document and alert the surgical support team to the need for specific protective measures for these patients.

The Association of peri-Operative Registered Nurses (AORN) has a—Prevention of Perioperative Pressure Injury—tool kit that is used in many surgical facilities. It has two tools that assist in the identification of at-risk patients. The Munro Scale tracks body mass index, body temperature, height, weight, and blood pressure. The Scott Triggers tool predicts at-risk patients based on their age, serum albumin, body mass index, American Society of Anesthesiologists score, and estimated length of surgery. These tools are limited in their effectiveness since they are determined on the day of surgery and do not allow adequate preplanning for positioning protective measures in the OR.

The Risk Assessment Scale for Perioperative Pressure Injuries (ELPO), developed and validated in Brazil, uses seven factors to predict patients at-risk for developing pressure injuries. (See table below). The ELPO Risk Assessment Scale is easily completed during the surgeon's pre-op visit and identifies issues that may impact patient safety during positioning of the patient for the surgical procedure. The surgeon or the surgeon's staff can submit the completed form with the orders for the surgical procedure. This provides the OR staff with information regarding special needs for positioning the patient on arrival in the OR. Examples of special needs include having an OR table designed for patients weighing more than 350 pounds and a HoverMatt for patient transfer when patients weigh more than four hundred pounds.

The surgeon's preoperative visit document should contain a statement that the patient having surgery is at risk for pressure-induced injury. The nature and significance of this type of injury were discussed with the patient and the patient seemed to understand and accept.

Even if special needs are identified preoperatively, time constraints may push perioperative team members to transport a patient to the OR before known preventive strategies can be implemented for the patient's protection.

Use of the edited ELPO form illustrated on the next page is a tool to reduce medical risk and facilitate preoperative planning for the surgical patient. A PDF copy of the form for your use is found in **Appendix A**. At the bottom of the form is a spot to indicate special equipment required for the patient's surgical procedure.

Patient Name: _____   Date of Surgery: _____   Surgeon: _____

Name of Surgery Facility: _____   Primary Procedure: _____

Date of Assessment: _____

ELPO Pressure Injury Risk Assessment Scale

Item \ Score	5	4	3	2	1	Value
Surgical Position	• Lithotomy	• Prone	• Trendelenburg	• Lateral	• Supine	
Surgery Duration	• Over 6 hr.	• More than 4 hr. Up to 6 hr.	• More than 2 hr. Up to 4 hr.	• More than 1 hr. Up to 2 hr.	• Less than 1 hr.	
Anesthesia Type	• General + Regional	• General	• Regional	• Sedation	• Local	
Support Surface: • OR Table • Limbs	• Thin pad • Thin or no pad	• Foam pad • Sheets or towels	• Foam pad • Foam pad	• Foam Pad • Viscoelastic pad	• Viscoelastic pad • Viscoelastic pad	
Limb Position	• Knees raised >90° • Lower limbs open >90° • Upper limbs open >90°	• Knees raised >90° • Lower limbs open >90°	• Knees raised <90° • Lower limbs open <90° • Neck without sternal alignment	• Upper limbs open <90°	• Anatomic position • Arms tucked palm to hip	
Comorbidities	History of: • Pressure ulcer • Neuropathy • Deep venous thrombosis	• Obesity (BMI > 35) • Malnutrition (BMI < 18.5)	• Diabetes Mellitus	• Vascular disease	• No comorbidities	
Patient age	• >80 years	• 70 to 79 years	• 60 to 69 years	• 40 to 59 years	• 18 to 39 years	
						Total Score:

Total score > 20 at increased risk for pressure induced injury.

Special equipment required in OR.

1.	4.	7.
2.	5.	8.
3.	6.	9.

Ref 3

Pre-Op Surgical Suite Room Review

Most surgical facilities store commonly used equipment in the surgical suite when the surgical suite is not being used. Different surgical suites may have different equipment stored in some of the non-sterile areas. If the surgical suite used for your surgery has the equipment you will be using for the day's surgery, your cases will proceed smoothly. If equipment needed for your surgery is not already in your assigned operating room (OR), you may incur delay during your surgery that interrupts your plan for your surgical case. Unanticipated starting and stopping of your surgical procedure disrupts your focus and may result in preventable unintended surgical errors. This unexpected procedure interruption is easily avoided by quickly inspecting the open non-sterile surgical suite assigned to your cases. In the non-sterile suite, you are looking for the proper table for your patient, the proper orientation of the table, the location of the lights and any monitors related to the position of the table in the room, and the appropriate energy sources and other equipment that will be used during your procedures.

The OR scrub tech assigned to your room for the day will usually be present in the room preparing for your first case when you come to the room. You can make your cases go smoother by asking the OR tech to obtain any items you notice are missing from the room. Likewise, if the room has an increased amount of equipment not used for your cases that day, you can ask to have some of the unnecessary equipment removed to prevent avoidable contamination of your surgical field. The diagram and table below are brief guides to help you survey room readiness for your surgical cases.

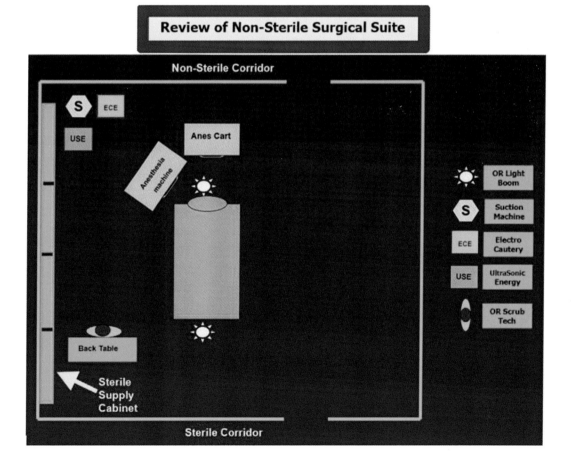

Pre-Operative Surgical Suite Checklist

- OR Table
    - Correct position for procedure
    - Appropriate size

- Adequate support equipment for the surgical team
    - Step Stools for team members
    - Rolling stool for surgeon when seated for procedure
    - Extra Mayo Stand for surgeon

- Standard OR Machines present and operational
    - Electrocautery machine
    - Forced-air patient warming device (Bair Hugger, and others)
    - Intermittent pneumatic compression device
    - Suction machine
    - Smoke evacuation machine

- Patient Transfer Methods
    - Lift sheet
    - Patient transfer board
    - HoverMatt
- OR Lights
- Video Monitors
- Specialty equipment
    - Laser
    - Imaging Equipment
    - Cell Saver
    - Video Cameras
    - Robot

OR Table

Correct Table Position

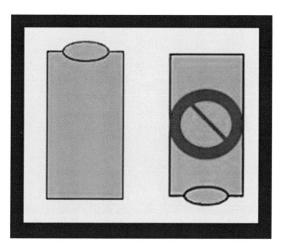

- The position of the OR table is significant to the safety of the patient. Make sure the head of the OR table is adjacent to the anesthesiologist. Occasionally, tables get turned 180° during the room-cleaning process, leaving the table in the wrong position for surgery. The head extension allows flexion of the neck and facilitates airway management by the anesthesiologist.
- Where does the table flex? Common areas where the table is segmented to allow flexion or extension include the neck, the thoracic-lumbar junction, and the hips. The patient needs to be positioned on the OR table to utilize these segmented areas optimally.
- Proper placement of the patient's hips over the leg board joint allows safe extension or flexion of the patient's legs. It is easier to make proper patient positioning before the patient goes to sleep.
- If intraoperative X-rays or C-arm visualization will be required, the OR table must have this capability. This can be determined prior to draping of the table, and the table can be exchanged before starting the case. **Not all OR tables have radiographic capabilities.**

Appropriate Size

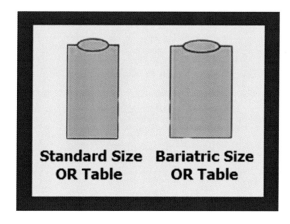

Standard Size OR Table   **Bariatric Size OR Table**

Not all OR tables can accommodate all sizes of patients.

- The standard OR table accepts patients up to **four hundred pounds.** The hydraulic lifts that raise and lower the table as well as change the tilt of the table have specific design limits. **Unpredictable failure can occur** if the patient's weight exceeds these limits. If this occurs during a surgical procedure, serious preventable injuries can occur.

- **Bariatric OR tables are designed for patients weighing more than four hundred pounds.**
  - These tables are wider.
  - The hydraulic lifts are designed to handle weights up to **one thousand pounds.**

Support Equipment for the Surgical Team

Step Stools

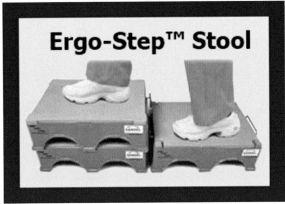

Ref 4

- The surgical team may have members of different heights. The OR table needs to be adjusted to create the best height for the active participants in the procedure (Surgeon, Assistant Surgeon, and Scrub Tech).
- The table height is adjusted so the tallest team member is standing comfortably on the floor. The efficiency of the surgical team depends on all team members being -ergonomically- comfortable and efficient during the surgical procedure. **This should be considered essential by the primary surgeon.**
- Step stools need to be provided for all other team members to reach the same height comfortably and safely. Occasionally, stools may need to be stacked.

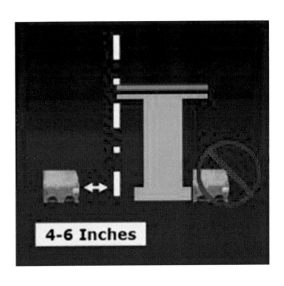

4-6 Inches

- The step stools should be four to six inches away from the OR table edge to allow ergonomic positioning for each member standing on step stools.

- If the **step stools are too close to the table**, the team member will have to stand on an unstable platform and use active energy to hold their arms close to their body, which may cause muscle fatigue and awkward movement.

Rolling Stool

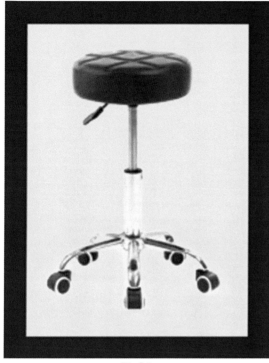

Ref 5

- When the primary surgeon is seated for the surgical procedure, the rolling stool height should be adjusted to create ergonomic efficiency for all team members. This may require the surgeon to use a step stool for their feet since the surgeon's stool height may not allow their feet to touch the floor if the assistant surgeon is tall.
- Older versions of the rolling stool screw the seat up and down to adjust the sitting height. Newer versions use a lever and a pneumatic assist to raise or lower the sitting height. Much easier!
- The benefit of having a rolling stool for the surgeon is that the wheels allow easy readjustment of the surgeon's position while remaining seated on the stool.
- Roller wheels should allow easy movement (i.e., not contaminated by residue from prior cases).
- Using the step stool for the surgeon's feet prevents compression irritation on the posterior aspect of the surgeon's thighs.
- The above recommendations allow the surgeon to maintain an ergonomic working position despite the height of the surgical assistant.

Extra Mayo Stand

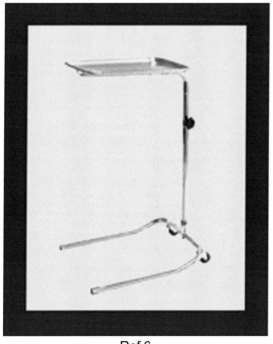

Ref 6

- During many surgical procedures, the surgeon may use several instruments repeatedly. While the surgical tech is responsible for keeping track of the instrument flow to and from the surgical field, strict adherence to this practice may slow the efficient progress of the procedure.
- Having an extra Mayo Stand convenient to the surgeon for the few instruments required repeatedly allows the surgical tech to focus on providing other necessary instruments timely when needed.

Standard OR Machines

Electrocautery

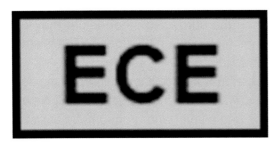

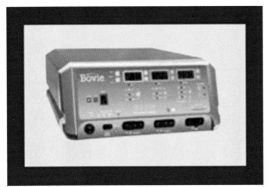

Reference 7

- Most electrocautery generators will provide both monopolar and bipolar current output.
- Monopolar current **requires grounding of the patient** with a special pad attached to the patient and **connected** to the machine.
- Inadequate grounding of the patient may result in unanticipated electrical burns in body cavities or on the skin surface in contact with the OR table when monopolar current is used.
- Bipolar instruments complete the electrical circuit between the tips of the instrument in contact with patient tissue.
- Use of bipolar energy avoids distant electrical burns.
- The tip of the instrument gets hot when used, and if the tip touches other tissue and remains in contact with the tissue, an unanticipated thermal injury may occur.
- The surgeon needs to understand the associated injury risks and minimize their occurrence when using electrocautery during a procedure.
- Surgical team members also need to recognize these risks and minimize these risks as they assist the surgeon.

Intermittent Pneumatic Compression Device

During a prolonged surgical procedure, patients with lower extremities fixed in an immobile position are at increased risk for thromboembolic events.

- One technique designed to decrease this risk utilizes a pump-and-sleeve combination to create intermittent tissue compression in the immobilized extremities, resulting in movement of blood through the veins back to the heart.
- Foot and Calf sleeves are commonly used.

Foot Sleeves

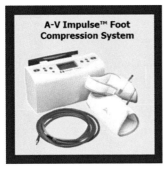

Ref 8

- **Foot sleeves are intermittent compression devices (ICD).**
- They create venous flow through-out the entire leg by compressing vessels in the foot.
- They are used when immediate post-op ambulation is desired since the patient can remove and replace the foot devices easily without assistance.

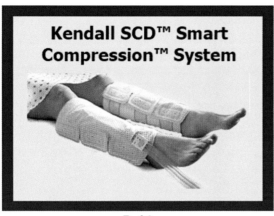

Kendall SCD™ Smart Compression™ System

Ref 9

- **Calf sleeves are sequential compression devices (SCD).**
- They have multiple compression compartments which move blood sequentially from the ankle to the knee.
- Blood flow created by this system is more physiologic, and fewer clotting issues are observed.
- The calf SCD requires assistance to remove and replace, resulting in less spontaneous post-op patient activity because personnel are not readily available to assist the patient.

Forced-Air Patient Warming Device

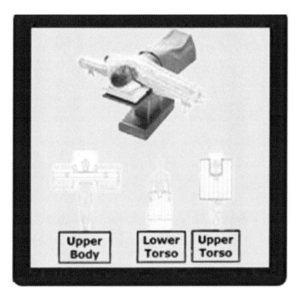

Ref 10

- General and regional anesthesia are frequently associated with decreased body temperature for many patients undergoing surgery.
- Hypothermia is associated with increased morbidity and mortality in the surgical patient. It is preventable.
- Forced-air warming systems are used to maintain body temperature in areas away from the surgical site.
- A common forced-air patient warming device found in many ORs is the Bair Hugger manufactured by 3M.
- The Bair Hugger provides warm air to different body areas as evidenced by the configurations illustrated in Figure 16.
- **While preventing the risk of hypothermia for the surgical patient, the warm air circulating around the patient and the operating table can increase the risk of airborne contamination of the surgical site.**

Suction Machine

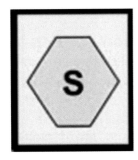

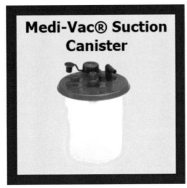

Ref 11

- Suction machines collect contaminated body fluids from the surgical field in disposable containers.
- Rather than using a specific machine that uses floor space, disposable fluid collection canisters attached to wall suction are used in many ORs.
- The containers are marked using metric volume measurements, allowing easy documentation of fluid loss from the surgical site.
- A chemical is placed in the disposable container at the end of the procedure to solidify the liquid contents and simplify management of the contaminated body fluids.

Smoke Evacuation Machine

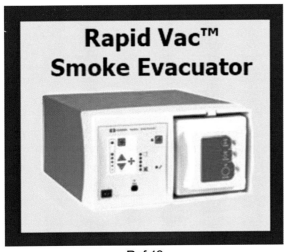

Ref 12

- Vaporization of body tissue during the use of electrocautery and laser devices results in smoke containing micronized tissue particles.
- When inhaled by members of the surgical team, adverse health conditions may occur.
- Smoke evacuation can be either a stand-alone machine with a sensitive filter or a central smoke evacuation system connected to the surgical site by a flexible tube. These systems are designed to remove a high percentage of particulate matter from smoke created at the surgical site.
- Not all particulate vaporized tissue is collected by smoke evacuator systems. If viral etiology is suspected for the tissue being vaporized, surgical team members should be wearing masks designed to filter viral particles from the surgical suite environment.

Patient Transfer Methods

Multiple reports in the literature conclude that **nurses have the highest occupational injury rate for back strain and pain of any industry or occupation.** Proper lifting techniques have reduced this injury risk in the OR setting. Several methods are discussed below.

- ## Lift Sheet

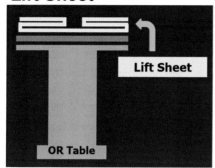

- The most common aide is the folded lift sheet placed under the patient at the time of surgery. It allows easy manipulation of the patient to change linens soiled during the procedure.
- It is occasionally used to lift patients from the OR table to the gurney. **Risk of back injury to staff using this method of patient transfer is high.**

- ## Transfer Board

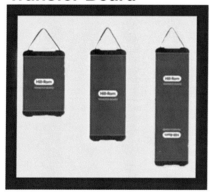

Ref 13

- The transfer board is the most common patient transfer method used in the OR.
- The transfer board is a light-weight, smooth, rigid material covered by a loose sleeve that slides over and around the board easily when a patient is placed on the board.
- Friction between the lift sheet and the cover of the transfer board caused by the weight of the patient allows the patient to slide across contiguous surfaces.

- ## HoverMatt

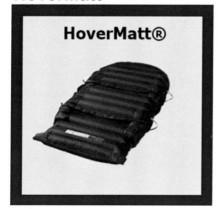

Ref 14

- The HoverMatt is a unique lifting device that allows high-pressure airflow to lift the patient and facilitate movement of the patient across a surface.
  - It reduces the force required for this movement by 80-90 percent.
  - **It significantly reduces the risk of back injury to caregivers in the OR.**
  - The unit can lift patients weighing as much as one thousand pounds and require only one person on either side of the mat to accomplish the task.
  - Single-use HoverMatts are also used today.
  - https://www.youtube.com/watch?v=jiC1sxBy9IY

OR Lights and Monitors

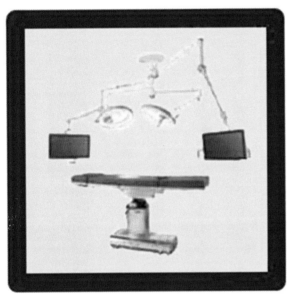

Ref 15

- **Ceiling-mounted lights**
  - o Arrange lights to focus on the approximate surgical field area prior to opening sterile instrument sets.
  - o Optimal surgical field illumination may require slight movement of the OR table.
  - o It is easier to move the OR table without a sterile-draped patient on the table.
  - o Risk of surgical field contamination by light adjustment is decreased when approximate light position is adjusted prior to patient positioning on the OR table.
  - o A primary cause of table-OR light maladjustment is table movement when the OR room is cleaned between surgical cases and the table is not returned to its functional position.

- **Ceiling-mounted monitors**
  - o Monitors are often used in the OR to allow team members better visualization of the surgical field.
  - o Monitor booms compete with OR lights for position around the surgical field.
  - o Boom-mounted monitors are positioned after OR light positions are established since the boom arms for the monitors may displace the boom arms for the surgical field lights.
  - o It is easier to adjust the monitor booms when the patient is not in the room.
  - o Verify the video camera system works on monitors to be used during the procedure. Signal connection cords are easily loosened over time, eliminating signal to the monitor.

Specialty Equipment

- Some equipment is used in nearly every surgical procedure and therefore is kept in most, if not all, OR suites.
- Confirming that necessary specialty equipment is present in the surgeon's OR for the day prevents interruption of the flow of the surgical procedure once the patient is anesthetized and draped.

Specialized Energy Sources

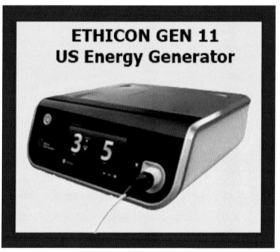

Ref 16

- Ultrasonic energy is frequently used for cutting and coagulation of tissue. In many instances, it replaces repetitive clamping, cutting, and suturing of tissue, resulting in significant shortening of the surgical time.
- The absence of this instrument in the room at the start of the case can significantly alter the course of the surgery if there is a delay in bringing the instrument to the room when it is urgently needed.

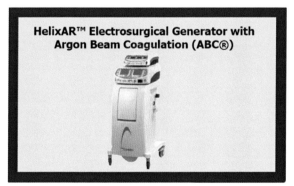

Ref 17

- The Argon Beam Plasma Coagulator uses a jet of ionized argon gas directed through a probe distant from the tissue target. Monopolar energy is conducted through the ionized argon gas coagulating the bleeding target tissue.
- Due to its unique usage profile, the Argon Beam unit needs to be in the OR at the start of the procedure.
- Sterile supplies necessary for its use should only be opened when the decision to use the Argon Beam coagulator is made.
- The absence of this instrument in the room at the start of the case can significantly alter the course of the surgery if there is a delay in bringing the instrument to the room when it is urgently needed.

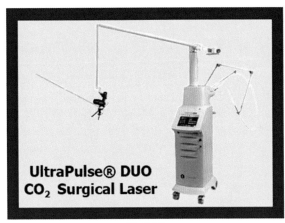

UltraPulse® DUO CO$_2$ Surgical Laser

Ref 18

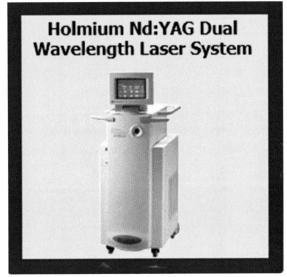

Holmium Nd:YAG Dual Wavelength Laser System

Ref 19

- Multiple lasers are now used for different surgical procedures.
- If one of these specific energy sources is scheduled for use in your case, confirm that the unit and its associated sterile disposable supplies are present in the OR suite before the case starts. ***Otherwise, significant surgical delays may occur.***
- •Sterile supplies necessary for the laser use should only be opened when the decision to use the laser is made. Otherwise, significant economic resources are wasted unnecessarily.

Imaging Equipment

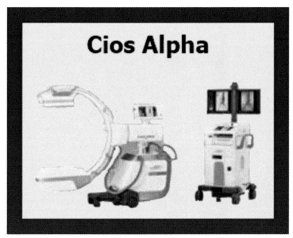

Ref 20

- Some procedures routinely need a C-arm during a portion of the procedure. Effective use of the C-arm requires an OR table designed for intraoperative X-rays. Not all OR tables are radiographic friendly.
- **Verify the OR table being used for your procedure is designed for radiographs if a C-arm is to be used during the procedure.**
- If the use of a C-arm is anticipated during the surgical procedure, request a room with a radiographic-capable table when the case is scheduled and request stand-by C-arm for the procedure.

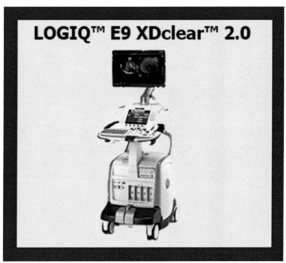

Ref 21

- Intraoperative Ultrasound requires unique transducers designed for the tissue to be scanned.
- Some of these transducers need to be sterile.
- Make sure the appropriate tissue transducers are present in the room before the case starts.
- Schedule the case for intraoperative Ultrasound Imaging to be available on stand-by for the procedure to ensure both the technologist and the equipment are available when needed.

Cell Saver

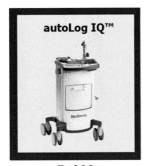

Ref 22

Video Cameras

- **External Mounted**
- **Endoscopic**
  - o **Flexible Scope**
  - o **Rigid Scope**

- **Robot**

  - o **Scopes**

  - o **Tools**

  - o **Drapes**

- Some surgical procedures are associated with excessive bleeding and loss of red cells. Cell savers are a machine that collects the patient's own blood cells, cleans them, and prepares them for reintroduction into the patient's vascular system, reducing the need for transfusion of blood-banked products.
- A specialized technician is required to operate this equipment and needs to be scheduled in advance when the equipment is scheduled for a case.

- Many OR suites have video cameras and monitors to improve visualization of the surgical site by members of the surgical team.
- Confirm that the cameras are functioning correctly and delivering images to the appropriate monitors prior to the start of the case.
- Endoscopic cameras should also be tested prior to the start of the case.
- If the video images are to be recorded, confirm that adequate recording space is available.
- Identify which surgical team member will be responsible for operation of the video system.

- Robotic surgery is currently used by many specialties, and set-up is considered routine.
- However, glitches may be avoided and set-up streamlined if certain issues are addressed prior to arrival of the patient in the OR.
- Confirm that the appropriate scopes are sterile and in the room. Some procedures require scopes of different diameters and/or lens angles for portions of the procedure. Not having these scopes sterile and in the room at the start of the procedure creates avoidable delays.
- Newer robotic video systems utilize a chip on the end of a flexible mechanical tube containing the electronics sending the image to the monitors.
- Confirm that all instruments are within their useful life. Most robotic instruments are designed for ten uses before they need to be replaced. Instruments having more than ten uses may not function properly and result in avoidable malfunction at critical times in the procedure.
- On occasion, specific drapes designed for a surgical procedure get contaminated. *Always* have an unopened sterile drape in the room to solve this problem if it occurs.

Pre-Op Review of the Surgical Suite

Preprocedure survey of the surgical suite can also be done as noted above. Since some of the sterile surgical instruments and drapes may be opened, all persons entering the room should be wearing masks and hair and shoe covering. The green areas in the diagram represent areas at increased risk for contamination of open sterile supplies and drapes. This is the time to note that necessary specialty equipment is present. If needed specialty equipment is not present, OR staff can retrieve the items to allow smooth progression of the surgical procedure. Some of the specialty equipment that may be necessary for the surgery is described in more detail below.

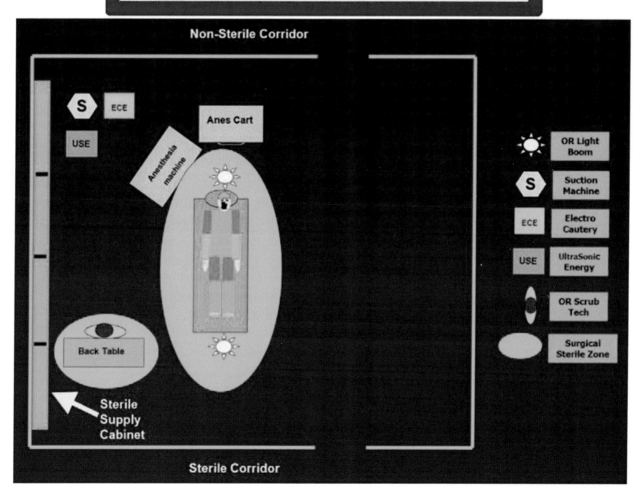

Sterile Supplies

- **Instrument Sets**
  - Routine Instrument Tray
  - Procedure Specific Tray
  - *Left-handed* Instruments
- **Retractors**
  - Routine
  - Specialty Retractors
- **Sutures**
  - Routine
  - Specialty

Instrument Sets

- **Routine instrument tray**
  - Facility specific. Contains all the sterile instruments necessary to support an emergency procedure.

- **Procedure specific tray**
  - Many instruments are uniquely designed to facilitate certain procedures. These specifically designed instruments are easily damaged if used inappropriately. Hence, they are often placed in separate procedure specific sets.

- **Surgeon preference cards**
  - Surgeon **procedure specific preference cards** stipulate when unique surgical sets and instruments are required.

- **Left-handed instruments**
  - **Having left-handed scissors and needle drivers available for left-handed team members significantly improves the ergonomic function of the surgical team.**

Retractors

- **Routine**

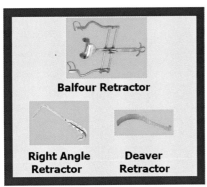

Balfour Retractor

Right Angle Retractor   **Deaver Retractor**

Ref 23

- Most standard abdominal instrument sets have a Balfour Retractor and numerous hand-held retractors included in the set.

Specialty Retractors

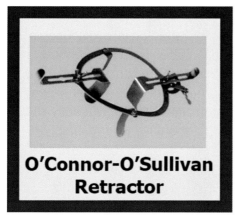

O'Connor-O'Sullivan Retractor

Ref 24

- The O'Connor-O'Sullivan retractor is a unique self-retaining retractor used in pelvic surgery to enhance exposure of the deep pelvic structures and to protect the bladder. All sides of the incision are retracted with equal force.

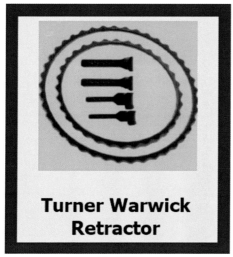

Turner Warwick Retractor

Ref 25

- The Turner Warwick retractor is another type of self-retaining retractor used in abdominal and kidney surgery. The tension of the retracted tissue holds the blades against the ring, creating the incisional retraction with equal force.

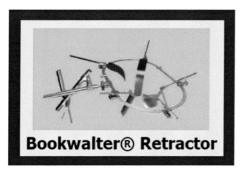

Bookwalter® Retractor

Ref 26

- The Bookwalter retractor is for large incisions and is securely attached to the side rail of the OR table. Malleable blades of different widths and lengths can be placed around the retractor ring to provide exact retraction as needed.

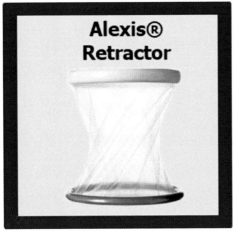

**Alexis®
Retractor**

Ref 27

- The Alexis retractor is a disposable retractor providing circumferential wound retraction while protecting the complete wound edge from drying out during the surgical procedure. The edge protection also significantly reduces the risk of postoperative wound infection.

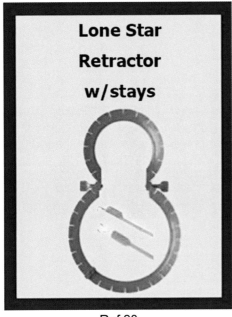

**Lone Star

Retractor

w/stays**

Ref 28

- The Lone Star self-retaining retractor is used in colorectal and gynecologic procedures. It is unique by using sharp, blunt, and curved retractor devices attached to stretchable tubing that can be placed in grooves anywhere around the circumference of the retractor. The ability to place specific retraction for the surgical field eliminates the need for a surgical assistant and the use of bulky instruments for the same task.

Sutures

- **Routine**

- **Special**

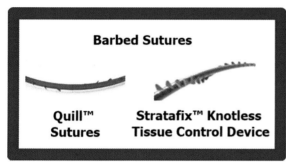

Ref 29, Ref 30

- o **Prolene, Gore-Tex, etc.**

- Surgeon preference cards normally indicate the preferred needles and sutures used for their procedures.
- Some procedures require unique sutures that have specific qualities.

- Barbed sutures are made of a synthetic absorbable monofilament with tissue absorption over an extended time. They do not need knots to secure the suture in tissue.
- The barb (cut in the suture) prevents slippage of the suture and maintains tissue approximation.
- Barbed sutures reduce tissue ischemia and necrosis by distributing tissue tension over the length of the surgical wound.
- Barbed sutures are not used to approximate structures that contain fluid under pressure (Bladder, bowel, blood vessels, ureter, etc.).
- Stratafix is unique in that it contains triclosan—a drug that inhibits methicillin-resistant S aureus (MRSA).

- Other applications require non-absorbable sutures that do not create tissue reaction. Prolene and Goretex amples.

Processing Patient in the Pre-Anesthesia Holding Area

After completing necessary sign-in formalities at the surgical facility on the day of surgery, the patient is escorted to the pre-anesthesia waiting area. At this point, the patient changes to appropriate clothing for the indicated surgical procedure. Certain steps are common to all surgical procedures and are discussed in more detail below.

Patient Preparation

Patient changes clothes

- Civilian clothes to surgical gown
- Wig/hair piece removed
- Hearing aids, glasses, and contact lenses removed
- Jewelry / body piercings removed

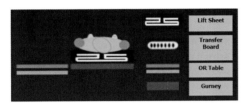

- The patient is lying on a folded lift sheet that will be used to assist in moving the patient to the OR table.

Receives Forced-air patient warming system

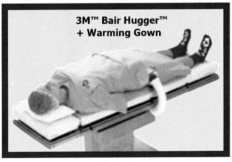

Ref 31

- Traditional patient gowns do not provide adequate coverage of the patient's skin surface, so body heat is easily lost. Once on the gurney, most patients receive a paper gown / blanket that plugs into a forced-air patient warming system that keeps them warm.

- ECG leads are placed in positions appropriate for their surgical procedure.

Place system monitors on patient

- Other monitors—Including pulse oximeter, blood pressure cuff, and intravenous line—are also placed.

- Pneumatic compression devices are placed on either the feet or calf.

Intermittent pneumatic compression device placed

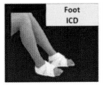 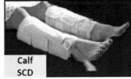

- Foot ICD intermittently compresses veins to force blood back to heart and relaxes veins to fill again.
- **Calf SCD** sequentially compresses veins from ankle to calf to knee to actually move blood back toward the heart. This method is more effective for clot prevention.

Meet Your OR Team!

The patient and their family members are anxious as they come to the surgical facility on the day of surgery. The only face they know is the face of their surgeon. Patient and family member anxiety is reduced when they know the people providing surgical care for the patient. When surgical team members introduce themselves to the patient and family members, anxiety levels decrease significantly. The normal surgical team members and their responsibilities are explained below.

OR Team Members

Each member of the surgical team has specific functions critical to successful completion of the surgical procedure.

Team members introduce themselves

- Studies have demonstrated that patient anxieties are markedly decreased when all members of the surgical crew working on their surgical procedure introduce themselves to the patient and their family.

Surgeon

- The surgeon is the individual responsible for bringing a person to the OR.
- The surgeon is the only familiar face of all the people the patient sees prior to the surgery.
    - The surgeon confirms the procedure to be performed and marks the surgical site.
- All activities occurring in the OR during a specific surgical procedure are ultimately the responsibility of the primary surgeon.

Anesthesiologist

- The anesthesiologist introduces themself and explains their role in the surgical procedure.
- The anesthesiologist is responsible for positioning the patient for the procedure and maintaining adequate airways and access to the vascular system.
- Induction of anesthesia and pre-induction assessment are also the responsibility of the anesthesiologist.

Other Members
• Anesthetist

- The anesthetist introduces themself and explains their role in the surgical procedure.
- The anesthetist monitors the patient during the surgical procedure. Maintaining an appropriate depth of anesthesia as well as appropriate fluid replacement and vital sign support are other responsibilities of the anesthetist.

- **Circulating Nurse**

  - During the procedure, the circulating nurse is the key contact person for the family until the patient arrives in the recovery room.
    - The circulating nurse asks the patient to describe in their own words the name of the procedure to be performed.
    - The circulating nurse also encourages the patient to ask any last-minute questions regarding the surgical procedure to be performed.
    - Communication to the waiting family with information related to the progress of the surgical procedure is another important function of the circulating nurse.
  - The circulating nurse is the person designated to manage all non-sterile activities that occur during a surgical case. These include retrieving additional sterile supplies, antibiotics, and blood products if needed.

- **Scrub Tech**

  - The scrub tech is responsible for pulling all the sterile supplies needed for the surgical case. Once they are present in the room, the scrub tech organizes the appropriate instruments on the sterile back table so they are readily available for the surgeon as the procedure progresses. The scrub tech also assists the other members of the surgical team to gown and glove in a sterile manner.

- **Surgical Assistant(s)**

  - One or more individuals may assist with the surgery.
    - The first assistant is normally a significant participant in the surgery, providing exposure for the surgeon and assisting with tying knots and cutting sutures.
    - Other individuals scrubbed in the case usually provide additional exposure of the surgical field for the surgeon.
    - These individuals may be
    - another surgeon or referring physician,
    - physician assistant,
    - nurse practitioner,
    - certified surgical assistant,
    - surgical resident in training,
    - medical student.

- **Observers in the OR**
  - **Medical students**

  - **Nursing students**

  - **Surgical tech students**

  - **Others**

    - **EMTs**

    - **Outside practitioners**

    - **Equipment representatives**

- Part of their education as they rotate through a service

- Part of their education as they rotate through a service

- Part of their education as they rotate through a service

- Others

  o Normally present to observe intubation techniques and airway management

  o Present to observe unique techniques to take back to their own surgical practice

  o Present to provide backup for implementation of new surgical tools and techniques

Transport to the OR

IV lines placed during the pre-anesthesia assessment allow anxiety-reducing medications to be administered to the patient prior to transport to the surgical suite. Most patients do not remember any of the happenings that occur from when they are moved to the OR until they awaken in the surgical recovery unit.

Medications Given for Transport to OR

- Reduce anxiety during transport
- Facilitate transfer of patient from gurney to OR table
- Decrease preinduction epinephrine surge
- Reduce arrhythmia risk

Transfer from Gurney onto OR Table

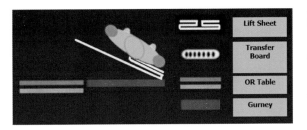

Patient Step 1

- Tilt the patient up and away from the direction of the transfer.
- Pull the lift sheet up and against the patient's back.

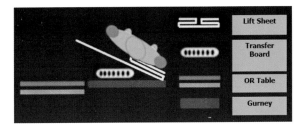

Patient Step 2

- Slide the transfer board between the lift sheet and the OR table.

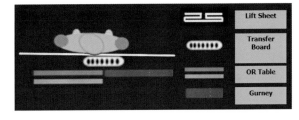

Patient Step 3

- Pull the lift sheet toward the OR table.
- Continue pulling until the patient is positioned completely on the OR table.

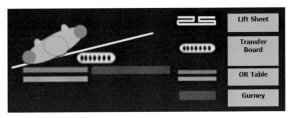

Patient Step 4

- Tilt the patient away from the gurney using the lift sheet.
- Remove the transfer board, allowing the patient to lie flat on the OR table.

Verify The Surgical Suite Is Ready Before the Patient Is Anesthetized

The patient is on the OR table. The OR scrub tech has sterile instruments and supplies open in the room. Other surgical team members are ready to position the patient. The Anesthesia team is ready for induction of anesthesia. This is the time for the Primary surgeon to confirm all necessary instruments, supplies, and specialty machines are in the room and ready for use if needed.

Once the confirmation is obtained, the surgeon gives permission for induction of anesthesia. **If intubation of the patient is required for the procedure, the surgeon commonly remains unscrubbed in the OR during the induction in case an unexpected anesthesia event occurs.** By remaining in the OR during the induction of anesthesia, a pair of skilled hands are immediately available for management of any unexpected anesthesia events. After induction of anesthesia is completed and the patient is properly positioned, the primary surgeon can leave the OR to scrub for the case. Other scrubbed and gowned members of the surgical team prep and drape the patient while the primary surgeon is scrubbing.

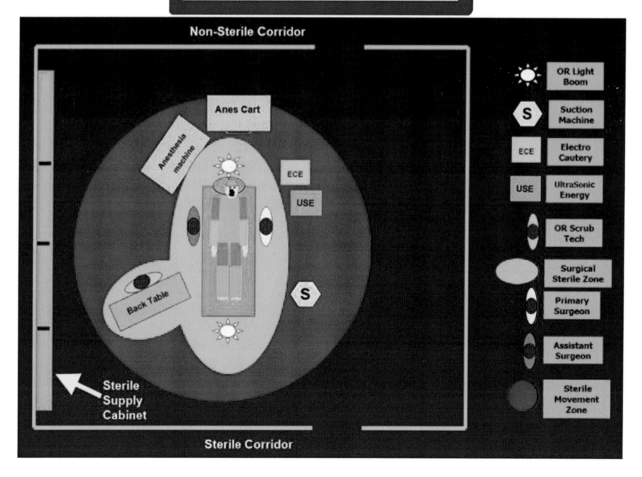

Sterile Surgical Suite with Surgical Team Ready for Surgery

Patient Positioning and Protective Padding

Padding

- During prolonged surgical procedures, tissue injury occurs due to compression and damage to underlying nervous and vascular structures.
- Risk of tissue injury may be reduced by using padding to cushion tissue at pressure points, such as
  - bony prominences and
  - foreign bodies held against the patient's body.
- Foam with some sponginess (i.e., egg—crate foam) should be used for padding and protecting soft tissue.
- **Sheets or surgical towels should not be used for padding.** They have no give and can create pressure injuries if used.

Most Common Surgical Positions

Supine Position

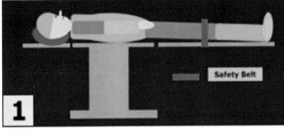
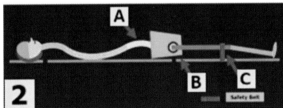
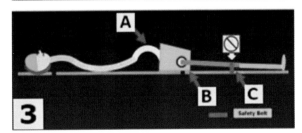

The supine or dorsal decubitus position is the primary position used in the operating room.

- While this position is easiest to perform, unintended issues occur when the patient is kept in the position for an extended period-of-time (greater than two hours).
- **(1)** Safety belt is **secure but not tight** to maintain normal pelvic rotation and keep legs from falling off OR table. The belt is located about two to three inches above the knee to provide optimal securing of the legs.
- **(2)** Illustration shows **(A)** normal lordotic curve of lumbar spine and **(B)** normal pelvic tilt in neutral supine position. **(C)** No under-knee support and safety belt is loose.

- **(3)** When the safety belt is tight the straight-leg position rotates the pelvis to the table. This causes extension of the lumbar spine, which may result in low back pain. **(A)** Increased lumbar curve extension is caused by posterior rotation of the pelvis. **(B)** The pelvis rotates posteriorly because of tight strapping of the leg in straight-leg position. **(C)** Tight Safety belt has no under-knee support.

Preferred Supine Position

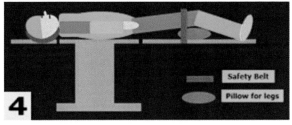

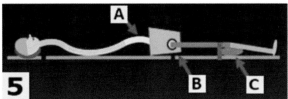

- **(4)** Placing a pillow under the knees reduces pelvic rotation and allows the lumbar vertebrae to maintain a neutral position.
- **(5)** Illustration reveals
    - o (A) normal lordotic curve of lumbar sacral spine,
    - o (B) normal pelvic rotation,
    - o (C) pillow under knee to maintain normal pelvic tilt and lumbar spine lordotic curve.

Arm Placement

Arms are either placed on arm boards or tucked adjacent to the patient's body, depending on the surgical procedure and/or the need for anesthesia to have access for monitoring the patient.

Arm Board Arm Placement

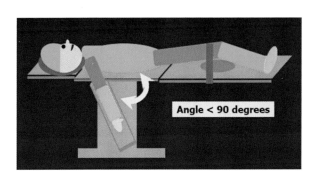

- When arm boards are used, the arm abduction should be less than ninety degrees.
- This position prevents excessive pressure of the humerus on the axilla from causing brachial plexus injury.
- Supination of the forearm with the palm down in the abducted position results in the least amount of pressure on the ulnar nerve, decreasing the risk of compression-induced ulnar nerve injury.

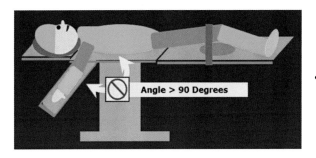

- When the arm abduction is greater than ninety degrees, the head of the humerus pushes into the axillary neurovascular bundle, possibly resulting in brachial plexus injury.

Arm Tucking

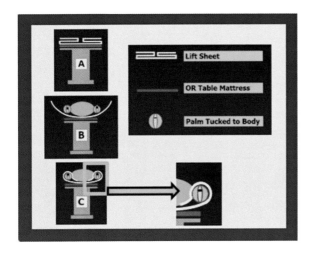

Tucking the arms adjacent to the body reduces nerve injury risk.

A. A lift sheet is fanfolded and placed under the thorax and abdomen.

B. The lift sheet is opened and extended under the arms.

C. It then encircles the arm to be tucked. The arms are tucked with the hand palm to the body and thumbs up. The remaining lift sheet is tucked securely between the patient and the OR table mattress.

This technique decreases external pressure on the ulnar nerve and minimizes injury risk to the ulnar nerve.

Inappropriate arm tucking increases the risk for brachial plexus injury.

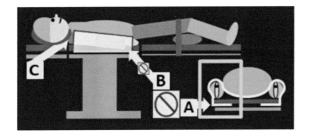

- **(A)** Lift sheet tucking arm between mattress and OR table. With the lift sheet in this position, it is easily dislodged, allowing the arm to fall from the table.
- **(B)** Hand and wrist are insecure and may easily flop off the mattress.
- **(C)** Shoulder pulled down by lift sheet between mattress and OR table, stretching brachial plexus nerves.

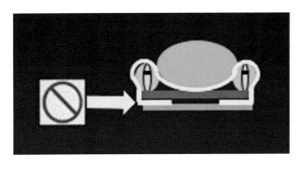

If the arm is tucked with the lift sheet between the body and arm and then over the arm and under the table mattress as illustrated, ***the sheet can work loose*** from its position, causing the arm to fall off the table, resulting in possible injury.

Leg and Heel Protection

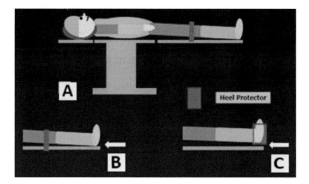

- **(A)** The figure shows a supine position with a straight leg and the heel resting on the bed. **(B)** The arrow points to the unprotected pressure point of the heel on the OR table.
- **(C)** Reveals the foam heel protector keeping the heel off the OR table and mattress.

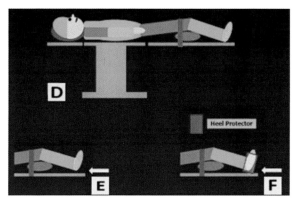

- **(D)** The heel presses on the OR table despite the knee being elevated by a pillow. **(E)** The arrow points to a pressure point.
- **(F)** The protective benefit of the foam heel protector keeping the heel away from the OR table surface.

Sequential Compression Devices (SCD) are frequently placed around the calf as prophylaxis for development of blood clots in the legs during long surgical procedures with patients in the supine position.

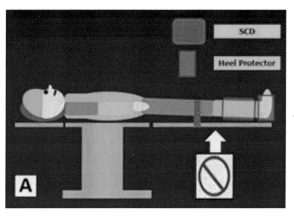 VS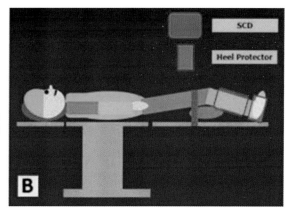

- **(A)** The patient is in the supine position with legs, calves, and feet flat on the table. The heel is protected by a foam heel pad. The calf has the SCD device surrounding it. The patient may develop low back pain caused by the prolonged extension of the lower back when the legs are flat on the table. **When in doubt, cushion the area behind the knees.**

- **(B)** shows the knees slightly flexed by a pillow. **The flexed knees allow the lumbar spine to maintain a neutral position during prolonged surgical procedures. A procedure is considered prolonged when the time the patient is on the OR table is greater than two hours.** This minimizes the risk of postoperative low back pain. **When in doubt, cushion the area behind the knees.**

Lithotomy—Supine—Candy Cane Stirrups

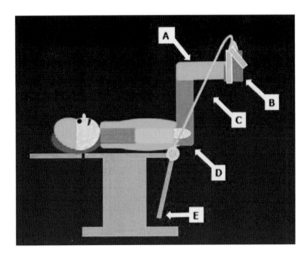

- The lithotomy position is commonly used in gynecologic, urologic, and colorectal procedures.
- **(A)** shows the leg parallel to the Thoraco-Abdominal axis. This position facilitates blood return to the heart from the lower extremities.
- **(B)** illustrates the foot protected by a foam cushion and attached to the Candy Cane stirrup pole with straps. The foam cushion protects the Achilles tendon.
- **(C)** illustrates the leg at a ninety-degree angle to the thigh.
- **(D)** shows the buttocks slightly past the end of the OR table. This positioning improves visualization of the surgical field by allowing soft tissue to fall away from the surgical field.
- **(E)** shows the foot board of the OR table folded greater than ninety-degrees to facilitate ergonomic positioning for surgical team members.

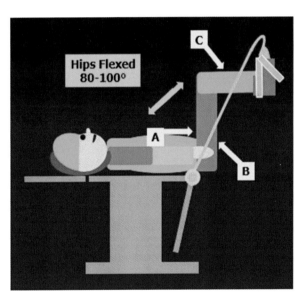

- The hips are flexed at eighty to one hundred degrees.
- **(A)** Flexion of the thigh more than one hundred degrees toward the abdominal wall increases the risk of femoral nerve compression and motor and sensory loss in the postoperative recovery period.
- **(B)** Obturator nerve injury also occurs with excessive flexion of the leg using Candy Cane Stirrups.
- **(C)** The leg should be parallel with the abdomen and thorax for proper positioning of the leg. This improves blood flow return from the lower leg.

Lithotomy—Trendelenburg—Candy Cane Stirrups

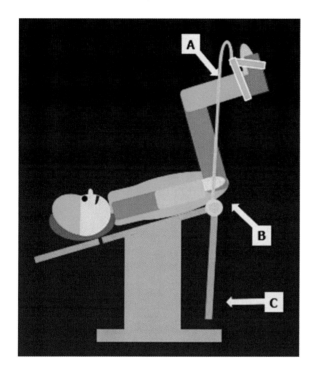

When the OR table is tilted in Trendelenburg position, the surgical team has **improved** visualization and **better** access to the surgical field.

- **(A)** shows the leg parallel to the Thoraco-Abdominal axis. This position facilitates blood return to the heart from the lower extremities. The Trendelenburg position of the table raises the heels and forces the thigh to rotate away from the surgical field. Rotation of the thigh away from the surgical field provides more space for ergonomic positioning of the surgeon and assistant surgeon.
- **(B)** shows the buttocks slightly past the end of the OR table. This positioning improves visualization of the surgical field by allowing soft tissue to fall away from the surgical field.
- **(C)** shows footboard of OR table folded greater than ninety-degrees to facilitate ergonomic positioning for surgical team members.

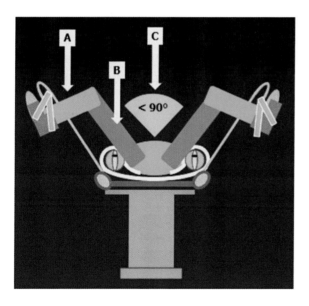

The perineal view of the patient in lithotomy position with candy cane leg supports is illustrated at the left. **Key points to consider include the following:**

- **(A)** Knee and calf need to be away from contact with the Candy Cane stirrup to avoid peroneal nerve injury.
- **(B)** The medial aspect of the thigh is at risk for pressure injury to the saphenous nerve if the assistant surgeon leans against the thigh for a prolonged time during the surgical procedure.
- **(C)** The thighs should be abducted at no more than a ninety-degree angle due to possible inadvertent injury to the hip joint or a stretch injury to the obturator nerve.

Allen Stirrups

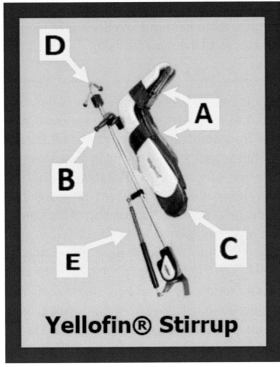

Yellofin® Stirrup

Ref 32

- The Yellofin stirrup is an improved version of the **Allen Stirrup,** which supports the foot and the calf on a pole away from the OR table. Other manufacturers produce similar leg supports with other names that perform the same function.
- **(A)** The stirrup provides a fixed protective position of the leg-foot angle.
- **(B)** Stirrup attachment allows movement of foot to obtain physiologic neutral positioning of extension of the thigh and lower leg.
- **(C)** The lateral fin is padded on the inside and protects the peroneal nerve and head of the fibula.
- **(D)** The lever allows change of elevation of the leg and change of external rotation of the leg at the hip joint to optimize neutral positioning of the leg during the surgical procedure.
- **(E)** The arrow identifies a mechanical spring assist for changing the up and down position of the leg.

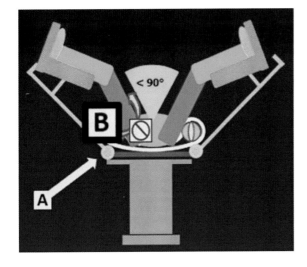

Allen Stirrups provide secure support to the calf and the foot. However, they are a bulky stirrup and impinge on the available space around the surgical field. The stirrup is designed to reposition the leg easily after the sterile surgical drapes are applied. *However, the ease of movement about the hip joint with Allen Stirrups increases the torque on the joint, risking unintended injury to the hip joint during surgery in the lithotomy position.*

- **(A)** The Allen Stirrup has a ball joint at the point where the stirrup attaches to the OR table. The ball joint allows the leg in the stirrup to be moved easier, increasing the risk of hip injury when adjusting the leg position to create more space for the surgical team.

- **(B)** *Excess* rotation of the Allen Stirrup at the hip joint increases the leg abduction angle greater than one hundred degrees creating increased stress on the hip joint.

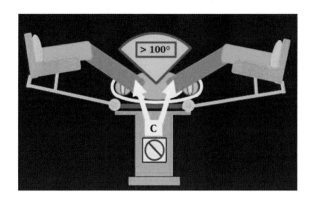

- **(C)** Point of increased stress on hip joint when angle between legs is greater than one hundred degrees.

Patient Position on OR Table in Lithotomy Position

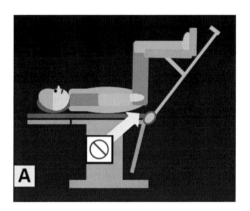

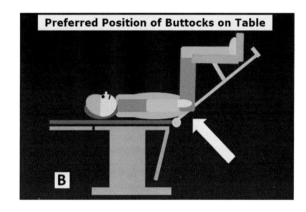

Figure A shows the patient with buttocks on the OR table (see arrow). This position creates issues when doing perineal surgery, including:

- compression of the perineal space, restricting visualization of the surgical field;
- restriction of the surgical field area, compromising effectiveness of instruments and tissue retractors;
- forces the surgeon to alter their surgical technique, leading to prolonged surgical time and increased risk for inadvertent tissue injury.

Figure B shows the patient with buttocks several inches off the OR table break (see arrow). With the buttocks off the table, the surgical field exposure is improved for the following reasons:

- Relaxation of the soft tissue around the buttocks drops tissue down and allows better retraction of the soft tissue away from the surgical site.
- The surgeon and the assistant have a better view of the surgical site, allowing the surgeon to work more efficiently with relaxed muscle tension.
- Less traction force is required to provide greater tissue exposure, resulting in less fatigue for the surgical assistant as well as the surgeon.
- Make sure the bottom edge of the table is well padded to protect the buttocks and sacrum from excessive pressure.

Other Examples of Common Lithotomy Positions

Lithotomy—Supine—Partial Leg Extension—Allen Stirrup

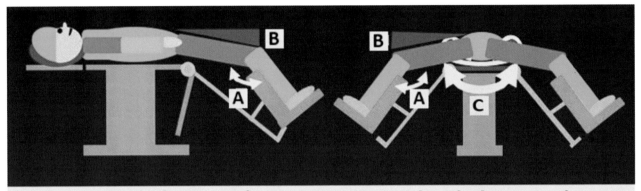

Supine Lateral View 150 degrees   Supine Perineal View 150 degrees

The above diagrams illustrate the lateral and perineal view of a patient using Allen Stirrups to support the lower extremities.

- **(A)** The 150° of leg extension provides a neutral position protective of hip, knee, and ankle joints; lower extremity nerves; and lower extremity blood supply.
- **(B)** Lowering the legs to position the thighs about 15° to 20° below the chest and abdomen increases space for a surgical team member adjacent to the patient.
  - o The perineal view with the thighs below the abdomen illustrates the enhanced ergonomic positioning for the second assistant between the legs.
- **(C)** Keeping the legs slightly below the line of the abdomen allows the stirrup rotation about the hip to remain in a neutral position. The angle of separation of the thighs is 100° to 110°. **If the leg was kept in the line of the abdomen, the 150° angle of extension would create excessive external rotation at the hip joint, resulting in pain and possible injury to the joint.**

Pearl: **Unrecognized joint injury caused by abnormal torque around the hip and/or knee joint can occur during positioning of the Allen Stirrups when the patient is anesthetized unless the above points are recognized and implemented.**

Lithotomy—Trendelenburg—Partial Flexion with Allen Stirrups

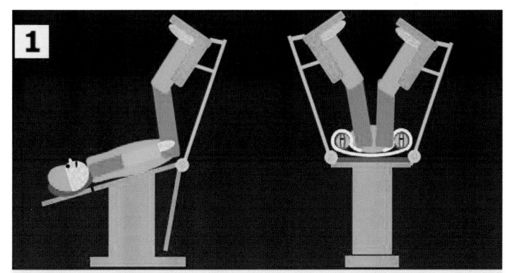

Trendelenburg Lateral View   **Trendelenburg Perineal View**

Figure 1 illustrates a lateral and perineal view of the patient in lithotomy position. The table is in Trendelenburg position at a twenty to thirty degree angle. The greater the angle of Trendelenburg position, the more pressure it takes to ventilate the patient. The legs of the patient are elevated at seventy to eighty degrees from the floor. This allows the surgeon and assistant to position themselves close to the surgical field. The legs are partially flexed at the knee in stirrups to relax tension on the nerves and improve blood flow return from the extremity to the heart.

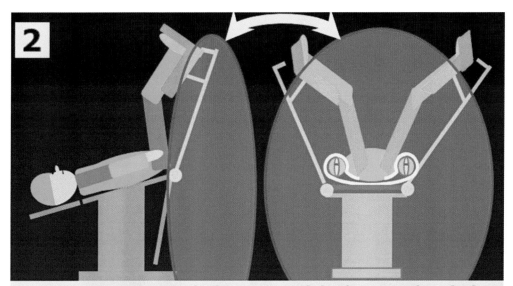

Trendelenburg Lateral View   **Trendelenburg Perineal View**

The yellow double ended arrow in **Figure 2** demonstrates how the Trendelenburg positioning with the legs elevated in stirrups maximizes the space for the surgeon and surgical assistant in perineal surgery.

Why Are Allen Stirrups Used?

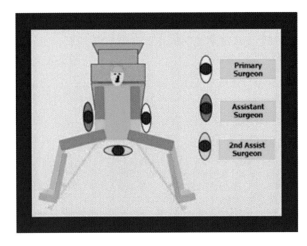

- To provide a more anatomic position for support of the legs during pelvic surgery.
- To avoid complications related to the calf, thigh, and hip.
- To provide a more secure positioning of the leg with less risk of pressure injuries.
- To provide a third space for an assistant in combined abdominal—pelvic procedures.

Allen Stirrups are particularly useful in training institutions where additional observers are frequently included in the surgical team.

Problems Related to Use of Allen Stirrups

- Allen Stirrups create less room for the surgical assistant adjacent to the perineal surgical field. The lack of space decreases the assistant's visualization of the surgical field, resulting in poor positioning of the assistant-held retractors and compromising the surgeon's surgical technique.
- When the surgical assistant leans over the thigh to assist the surgeon, increased pressure on the thigh may induce pressure-associated injury to underlying nerves.
- The Allen Stirrup increases risk of injury to the hip joint because repositioning of the leg for better visualization of the surgical field easily creates excessive external rotation and abduction about the hip joint, resulting in postoperative pain at the involved hip joint.

Trendelenburg Position—Supine

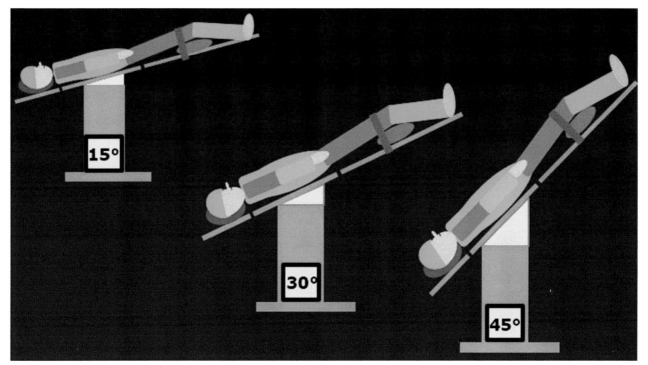

Ref 33

Trendelenburg position: A variation of supine in which the head of the bed is tilted down such that the pubic symphysis is the highest point of the trunk. It facilitates venous return to the heart. The head-down position allows gravity to pull the abdominal contents cephalad, improving pelvic cavity visualization during abdominal and laparoscopic surgeries. The Trendelenburg position is usually fifteen to forty-five degrees below level. **Steep Trendelenburg is considered thirty to forty-five degrees below level.** It is rare for patients to be positioned at angles greater than thirty to thirty-five degrees below level because of the increased risk of the patient sliding cephalad. Shoulder braces to prevent sliding when patients are in Steep Trendelenburg position are not used because of the increased risk of brachial plexus nerve injury that occurred with their use in the past.

Trendelenburg Position—Risk of Slipping

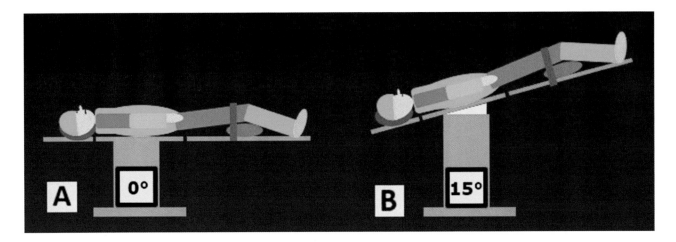

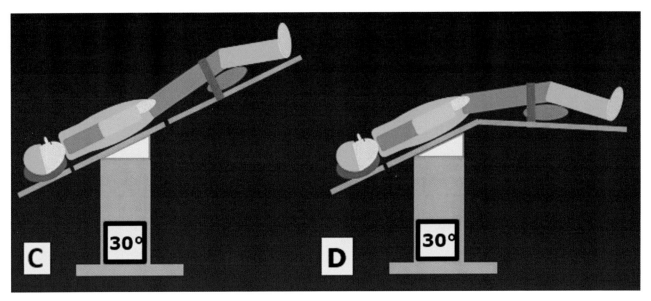

(A) **Zero-degree** Trendelenburg—No risk of slipping. Arms and legs need to be secured to prevent extremities from sliding off the OR table. Arms may be secured on an arm board or tucked adjacent to the body.

(B) **Fifteen-degree** Trendelenburg—**At fifteen degrees**—risk of slipping is increased about twice that of the supine position. A pillow under the knees with a secure strap over the thigh and secure tucking of the arms will minimize the amount of slipping observed during a surgical procedure.

(C) **Thirty degree** Trendelenburg—At thirty degree Trendelenburg, the risk of cephalad slipping is increased about five times greater than that seen with the supine position. A pillow under the knees and tucking of the arms does not change the risk of slipping at this degree of Trendelenburg.

(D) **Thirty degree** Trendelenburg with **ten degree extension** of the thigh. When the thigh is extended about ten degrees, the impact of the increased Trendelenburg angle is minimized and the risk of slipping is only about three times more than that of the supine position for the same degree of Trendelenburg.

Internal Organ Position Related to OR Table Position

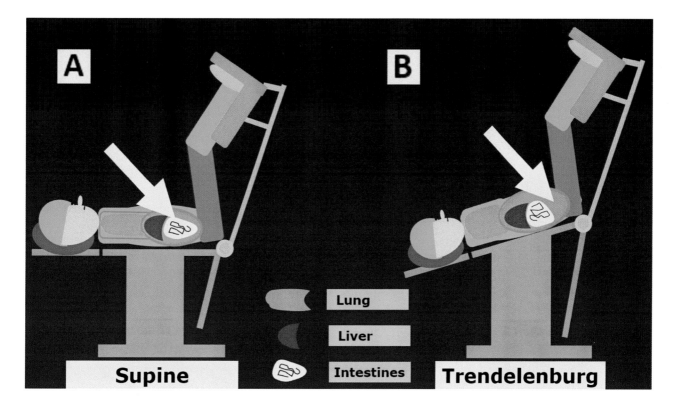

When operating in the pelvis, internal organs are frequently pushed into the operative field by respiratory diaphragmatic movement, complicating visualization of the focus point of the surgery. The above pictures illustrate the lithotomy position commonly used for pelvic/colorectal surgery.

Figure A shows the upper body in the supine position. In **A**, the lungs have normal volume and respiration is not anatomically restricted. The space surrounding the abdominal organs is minimal as indicated by the **arrow**. If the procedure is being performed through an abdominal incision, retractors and packing of tissue away from the surgical area of interest are commonly used to prevent intrusion of adjacent tissue into the surgical field.

Figure B shows the upper body in Trendelenburg position. The lung volume is decreased because of the impact of gravity, causing movement of the abdominal organs toward the diaphragm. Ventilation of the lungs is slightly more difficult because the weight of the abdominal organs restricts diaphragmatic movement. However, with the shift of the abdominal organs cephalad, the free space in the pelvis is increased as indicated by the **arrow** in diagram **B**. When the surgical procedure is being performed using minimally invasive surgical techniques, simply changing the body to Trendelenburg position will allow gravity to move the internal organs out of the way. The steeper the Trendelenburg position, the more operative space is created.

Many surgeons now use this technique in open abdominal cases as well.

Patients for abdominal surgery are commonly positioned supine with the legs straight and level with the thorax and abdomen.

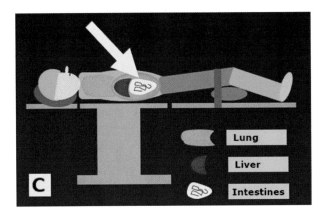

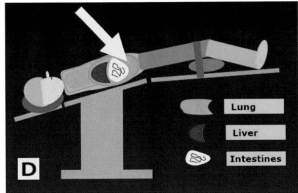

- When the patient is flat, as illustrated in **C**, the lungs function normally.
- The abdominal organs spread throughout the abdominal cavity.
- **Exposure of the surgical field requires mechanical force to keep the surgical incision open.**
  - Mechanical retractors can be locked in place at the desired opening.
  - Handheld retractors depend on the strength and attention of the surgical assistant holding the retractor.
  - If the assistant's attention to the operative field changes, the retraction can suddenly decrease, impairing the surgeon's view of the operative field. Unintended consequences can occur.
- Surgical packing with moist, soft material can also prevent bowel and omentum from moving into the surgical field inadvertently.

- **The benefits of Trendelenburg position for open abdominal procedures** are readily recognized by comparing **Figure C** with **Figure D.**
  - The abdominal organs shift toward the diaphragm, decreasing the amount of tension required to expose pelvic surgical fields.
  - The need for surgical packing is reduced or eliminated for the same reason.
- By slightly extending the thigh at the hip joint and securing the leg with the safety strap above the knee, the risk of movement of the patient cephalad by sliding down the table is reduced.

Post-Op Pain Caused by Gas Trapped in Diaphragmatic Space between the Liver and the Diaphragm

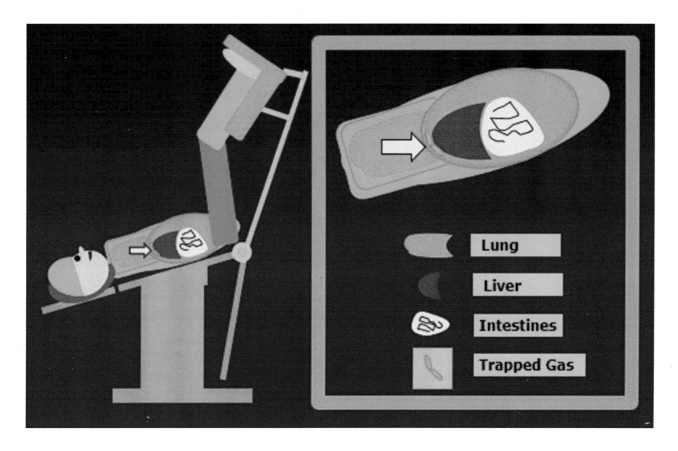

CO_2 is the gas used to distend the abdomen in laparoscopic surgical procedures. **The CO_2 gas is normally absorbed through the peritoneum into the blood circulating in the vascular system and removed through the lungs within twenty-four to forty-eight hours.** Intraperitoneal gas is usually infused with the patient in the supine position and released with the patient in the Trendelenburg position. In the supine position, the hepato-diaphragmatic space is slightly increased because the liver rotates caudally and away from diaphragm. The Trendelenburg position can trap gas bubbles between the liver and the diaphragm (bubbles like Bubble Wrap) when the liver rotates back against the diaphragm. Unless the trapped gas is displaced prior to the end of the procedure, respiratory movement of the diaphragm may result in pain referred to the epigastric/substernal area, which will persist until the CO_2 gas is absorbed.

Post-op pain may be prevented by displacing gas trapped in the diaphragmatic space between the liver and the diaphragm with irrigation fluid.

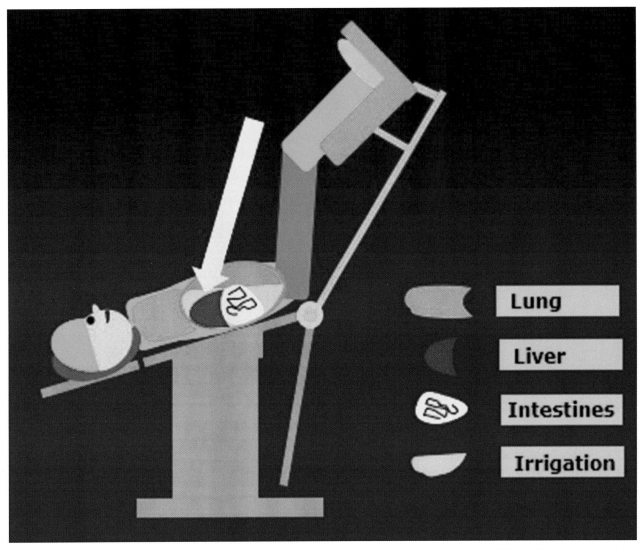

CO$_2$ gas trapped in the hepato-diaphragmatic space can be minimized by filling the space with irrigation fluid (usually 300—500 ml of normal saline solution) until the fluid level is above the dome of the liver before returning the patient to a neutral position. After irrigation solution has filled this space, the patient position may be returned to the supine position. Surface tension between the diaphragmatic surface and the dome (arrow) of the liver will maintain a thin film of fluid and prevent gas from causing referred pain. By displacing trapped gas from this space with normal saline irrigation solution, postoperative substernal pain is frequently eliminated or minimized.

Irrigation fluid, such as normal saline solution, is absorbed into the vascular system through the peritoneum. The excess fluid is removed by the kidneys. Residual fluid between the liver and the diaphragm displaces trapped pneumo-peritoneal gas and allows the normal buffer between the surface of the liver and the diaphragm to reform without the pain-causing trapped bubbles of gas.

Physical and Physiologic Changes Associated with Trendelenburg Position

Physical Changes

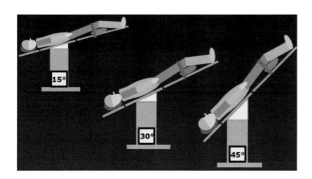

- **Steep Trendelenburg position**

  - o **Thirty to forty-five degrees**

- **Prolonged OR time**
  - o **Greater than two to three hours**

When both conditions above are present, changes may occur in the following:

- **Upper airway and head**
  - o Increased intracranial pressure
  - o Increased intraocular pressure
  - o Swelling of the face, larynx, and tongue with possible postoperative airway obstruction due to edema
  - o Periorbital edema may occur. It is usually short-term and leaves no residual injury.
  - o Edema clears with normal supine position post-op.

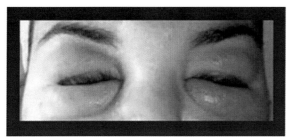

Ref 34

Physical Changes (continued)

- **Body may slide cephalad. Prevented by the following:**

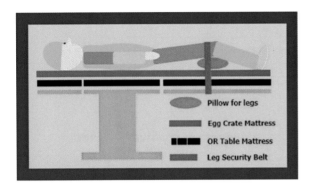

- Egg-crate foam mattress between the patient and the OR table mattress.

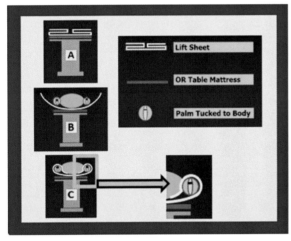

- Tight tucking of the arms against the body

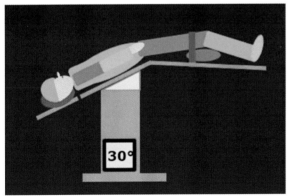

- Slight flexion of the leg board

Physiologic Changes

- **Hemodynamic changes**
  - Increased venous return
  - Increased cardiac output
  - Temporary related to intraoperative and immediate post-op time in Trendelenburg position.
  - Majority of changes return to baseline within minutes of return to supine position

- **Respiratory changes**
  - **A-1** Normal lung with normal functional residual capacity.
  - **A-2** Normal position of liver against the diaphragm in the supine position.
  - **B-2** Trendelenburg position moves abdominal contents toward the diaphragm in a cephalad direction.
  - **B-1** Trendelenburg position decreases lung volume resulting in
    - decreased functional residual capacity and
    - decreased respiratory compliance.
  - These changes are managed by ventilation with higher airway pressure.
  - These changes resolve quickly with return to the supine position.

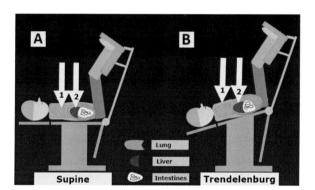

49

Reverse Trendelenburg

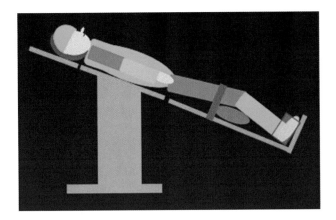 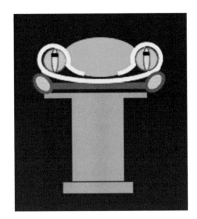

Reverse Trendelenburg positioning is frequently used for surgical access to the upper abdomen. A foot board is securely attached to the table to support the patient's body weight. The legs must be secured to the table with a wide strap about three inches above the knees. As with other body positioning, the knees must be protected from hyper-extension by placing a pillow posterior to the bend of the knee. The heel should be protected by a foam cushion.

- The arms should be tucked by the patient's side using a lift sheet that passes under the patient's body and encircles the arm. The end of the lift sheet is tucked tight and secure under the patient's body.
- Foam padding should be placed under the elbow and arm before tucking the arms to protect the nerves from excessive pressure during the procedure.
- If the arms extend over the edge of the table on either side, add an arm board parallel to the table to provide additional support for the tucked arm.

How to Increase Upper Abdominal Space with Reverse Trendelenburg Position

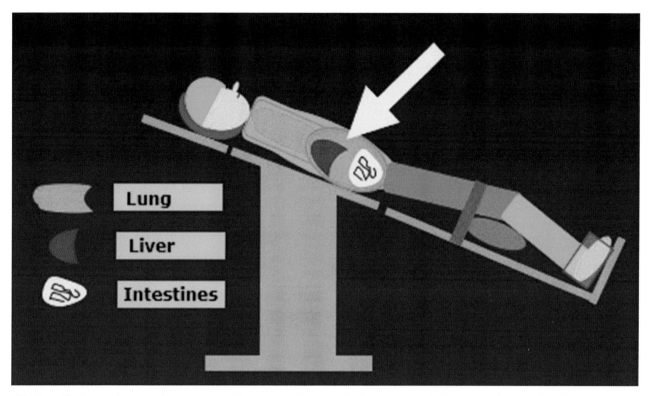

Notice that gravity produces some increased space in the upper abdomen when using the reverse Trendelenburg position by using the weight of the omentum to drop it into the pelvis.

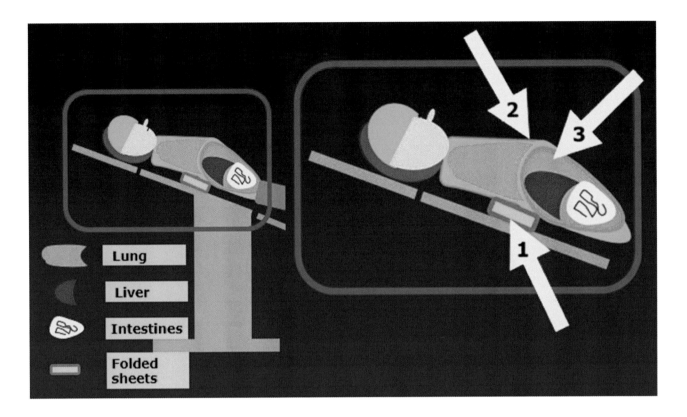

Using folded sheets under the lower thoracic spine increases upper abdominal space further.

(1) Two or three folded sheets placed under the lower thoracic spine cause the upper thoracic spine to extend.

(2) The thoracic ribs rotate open, resulting in a larger antero-posterior diameter at the level of the sternum.

(3) The surgical space in the upper abdominal cavity is increased in volume, facilitating surgical manipulation of the tissue in this area.

Impact of Position on Spinal Curves

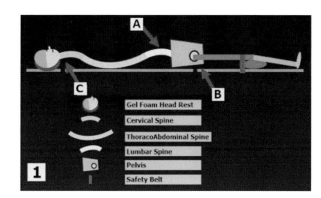

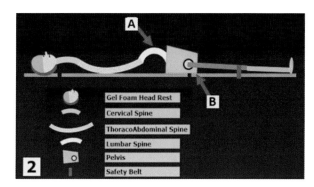

Spinal curve orientation for normal patient position on OR Table

- **(A) Slight flexion of lumbar spine**
- **(B) Normal pelvic tilt maintained by under-knee support**
- **Cervical and Thoraco-Abdominal spine curves maintained**
- **(C) Gel foam doughnut under head to prevent excessive extension of the cervical spine during the surgical procedure**

Lack of under-knee support

- Flattens thigh.
- **(A)** Increased Flexion of the Lumbar Spine straining intervertebral spaces.
- **(B)** Results in loss of pelvic tilt.
- May cause significant low back pain in post-op recovery state.
- These issues apply to all age groups but may be more pronounced in older individuals.

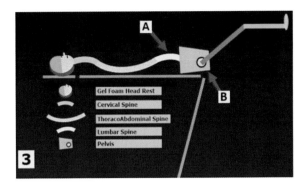

Lumbar Sacral Spine protected with proper leg support

- The stirrups must be adjusted to maintain normal lumbar curvature **(A)** and normal pelvic tilt **(B)** during perineal procedures.
- Maintaining the proper pelvic tilt is necessary to minimize excessive flexion or extension of the lumbar spine.

The stirrups (candy cane or Allen) are not illustrated in this diagram to allow clear demonstration of the anatomic position of the spine, legs, and pelvis.

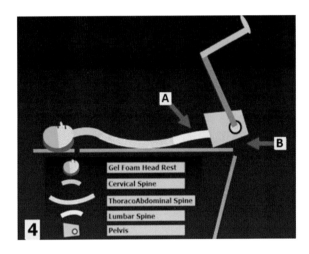

Excessive leg flexion impact on Lumbar Sacral Spine

- **(A) Excessive flexion using either candy cane or Allen stirrups will alter the pelvic tilt and result in extension (flattening) of the lumbar spine.**
- **(B) Notice the pelvic angle is increased away from the OR table.**
- **Low back pain as well as sciatic pain may be observed when this position occurs.**

The stirrups (candy cane or Allen) are not illustrated in this diagram to allow clear demonstration of the anatomic position of the spine, legs, and pelvis.

OR Table Positions for the Surgical Team

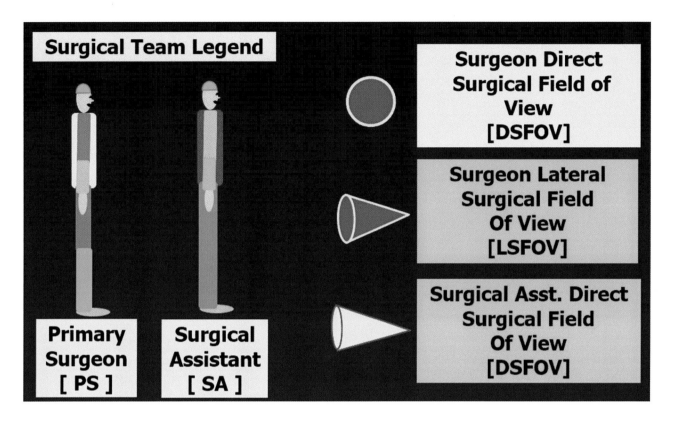

The primary surgeon **(PS)** is responsible for the patient's surgical outcome.

- The **PS** directs positioning and job function for all other members of the surgical team.
- The **PS** determines the most appropriate patient position for the surgical procedure.

The Surgical Assistant **(SA)** is the surgical team member responsible for enhancing the surgical field of view.

- Depending on the surgical procedure, the **SA** may be a:
  - Physician,
  - surgical resident,
  - physician assistant,
  - nurse practitioner,
  - certified OR tech,
  - student.

- The Surgeon's Direct Surgical Field of View **(DSFOV)** is the view the surgeon has when looking straight ahead with a relaxed position of the surgeon's head.
  - The primary operational field of view is encompassed in a thirty-degree cone centered on a line from the surgeon's eyes to the center of the surgical field.
- The Surgeon's Lateral Field of View **(SLFOV)** is represented by the *blue* cone.
- The Surgical Assistant's **DSFOV** is represented by the *yellow* cone.

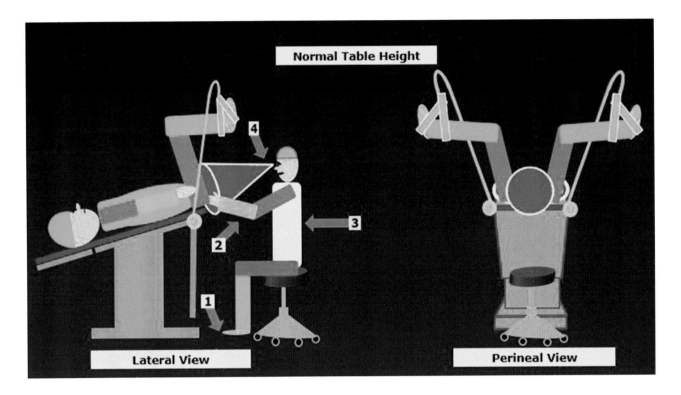

Normal Table Height

Lateral View

Perineal View

(1) illustrates the Normal Table Height and has the surgeon sitting on a stool with both feet on the floor.

(2) demonstrates the surgeon's position away from the surgical field to allow the elbows to be comfortably bent. (i.e., not fixed and locked straight!).

(3) illustrates the ergonomically straight surgeon's back. Any forward leaning of the surgeon's back increases muscle fatigue and adds stress and muscle tension as the duration of the procedure increases.

(4) illustrates the ergonomic angle of the surgeon's field of view. The line from the surgeon's eyes to the center of the surgical field is about fifteen to twenty degrees below the horizon.

In the perineal view illustrated above, the surgeon's field of view is the blue circle correlating with the base of the cone shown on the left.

Surgical Assistant Positions with Abdominal Surgery

Overhead View with patient in Supine Dorsiflexion Position

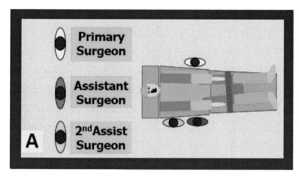

Right-handed surgeon with
a pelvic surgical field

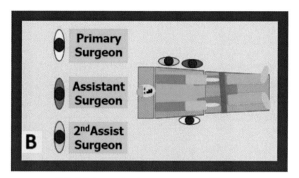

Right-handed surgeon with an
upper abdominal surgical field

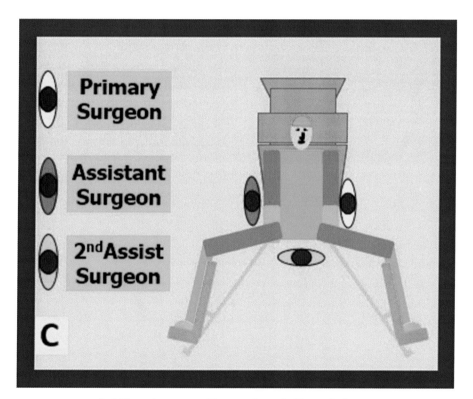

Lithotomy Surgical Position
Right-handed surgeon with a *pelvic surgical field*

(A) This diagram illustrates the usual surgical team positions for a right-handed surgeon with a surgical field in the pelvis. The Assistant is usually across from the surgeon.

(B) When a right-handed surgeon is working in the upper abdomen, the positions are frequently flipped.

(C) This figure illustrates the surgical team positions for a right-handed surgeon using a pelvic surgical field with the patient in a lithotomy position.

Surgical Assistant Position—Lithotomy Using Candy Cane Stirrups

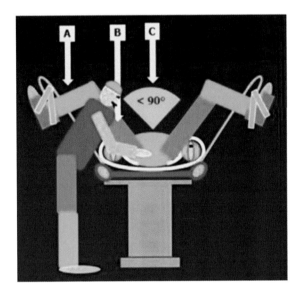

- Injury to the common peroneal nerve is the most frequent pressure-induced nerve injury for patients having surgery in the lithotomy position. While low BMI and prolonged surgical times are suggested as the main factors associated with its occurrence, a more likely cause is inadvertent pressure on the leg caused by the surgical assistant attempting to get a more ergonomic stance during the surgical procedure.
- **(A)** Minimal shifting of the assistant surgeon posteriorly can initiate contact between the assistant surgeon and the calf of the patient, pushing the calf against the Candy Cane stirrup, resulting in peroneal nerve injury.
- **(B)** Minimal shifting of the assistant surgeon cephalad can initiate contact between the assistant surgeon and the thigh of the patient, creating a pressure-induced injury to the saphenous nerve.
- **(C)** Minimal shifting of the assistant surgeon cephalad can also force the hip to abduct greater than ninety degrees, exacerbating pre-existing arthritic disease of the hip.

Surgical Assistant Position—Lithotomy Using Allen Stirrups

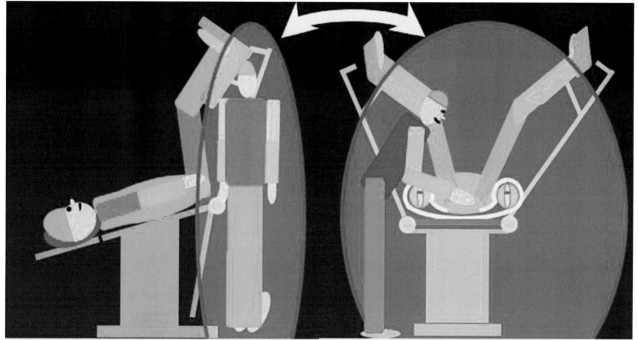

Trendelenburg Lateral View   **Trendelenburg Perineal View**

In the lateral lithotomy view above, the right leg and associated Allen Stirrup are not shown to better demonstrate how the Allen Stirrups should be positioned. The illustration demonstrates the ability of the surgical assistant to be immediately adjacent to the flexed patient leg, facilitating the assistant's ability to visualize the surgeon's field of view as well as provide adequate exposure for the surgeon.

The perineal lithotomy view illustration confirms the surgical assistant's (SA) ergonomic position of the arms, back, and legs. By allowing the SA to maintain an ergonomic position, the SA will minimize development of positional fatigue during the surgical procedure.

Alternative Surgical Assistant Position—
Lithotomy Using Allen Stirrups

The primary function of the surgical assistant is to provide optimal visualization of the surgical field for the surgeon. This requires the surgical assistant to have a position to retract tissue and suction the surgical field. This is best accomplished when the assistant stands adjacent to the surgeon between the legs of the patient in the lithotomy position.

- When Allen Stirrups are used for the lithotomy position, the assistant surgeon frequently must stand outside the legs of the patient. **This places the patient at risk for several unintended events.**

- **(A)** The assistant frequently must stand on a stool to create adequate reach to the surgical field.
    - o This posture is ergonomically unstable.
- **(B)** Provision of adequate retraction for the surgeon by the surgical assistant may:
    - o place excessive pressure on the medial thigh, resulting in sensory loss involving the femoral nerve;
    - o create a pressure-induced injury to the lateral aspect of the leg below the knee, involving the lateral peroneal nerve;
    - o need readjustment of the Allen Stirrup to a better position, creating abnormal stress on the associated hip joint.
- **(C)** The surgical assistant may be physically unable to visualize the surgical field, resulting in compromised visualization of the surgical field for the surgeon, yielding:
    - o prolonged surgical time due to frequent readjustments of retractors to optimize visualization of the surgical field and
    - o increased risk for inadvertent tissue injury.

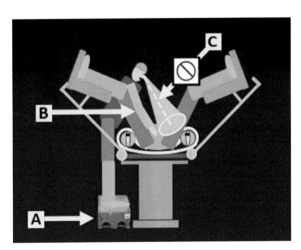

Optimizing Short Surgical Assistant Position—Lithotomy Using Candy Cane Stirrups

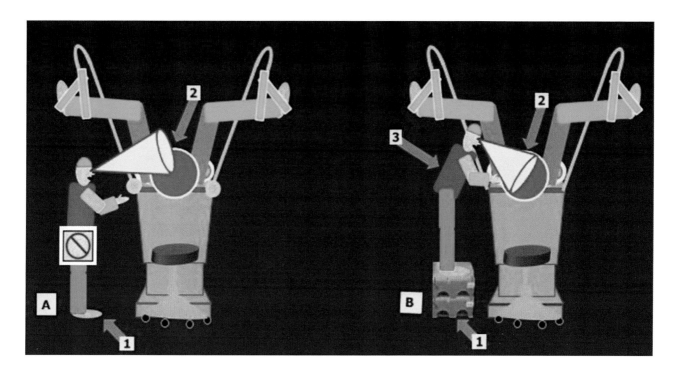

(A) Picture shows perineal view with the table set at the normal height for the primary surgeon **(PS)**. A short surgical assistant **(SA)** is positioned next to the surgeon's stool.

- o **(1)** shows the **SA** with feet on the floor.
- o **(2)** demonstrates the **SA** ergonomic field of view above the **PS** field of view.
- o **This position compromises the PS's ability to utilize the SA and leads to increased tension and fatigue for the SA.**

(B) solves the positioning problems for the short **SA** and the **PS** by using stools for the **SA**.

- o **(1)** raises the height of the **SA** to the level of the **PS**.
- o **(2)** illustrates the fact that the **SA** field of view is the same as the **PS** field of view. This results in improved efficiency for both the **PS** and **SA**.
- o **(3)** illustrates ergonomic positioning of the **SA's** back, reducing **SA** back muscle tension and fatigue during the surgical procedure.

Tall Surgical Assistant Challenging Position—
Lithotomy Using Candy Cane Stirrups

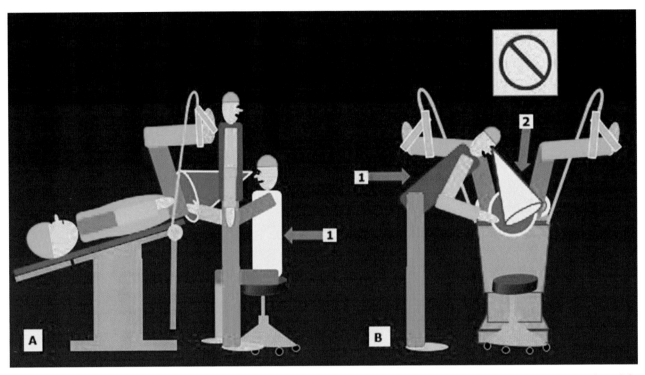

(A) Normal table height for the primary surgeon **(PS)**

- Note that the **PS** has feet flat on the floor and **(1)** the back of the **PS** is ergonomic.
- The **PS** field of view is also ergonomic.
- The *tall* surgical assistant **(SA)** standing straight has his/her head above the patient's feet.

(B) shows why this position should not be used.

- The surgeon's position has not changed.
- **(1)** shows the **SA's** back is excessively forward flexed, resulting in increased muscle tension and accelerated fatigue.
- **(2)** illustrates the **SA** field of view slides away from the surgeon's field of view, compromising the **PS's** surgical efficiency and increasing risk for adverse events.

Tall Surgical Assistant Optimal Position— Lithotomy Using Candy Cane Stirrups

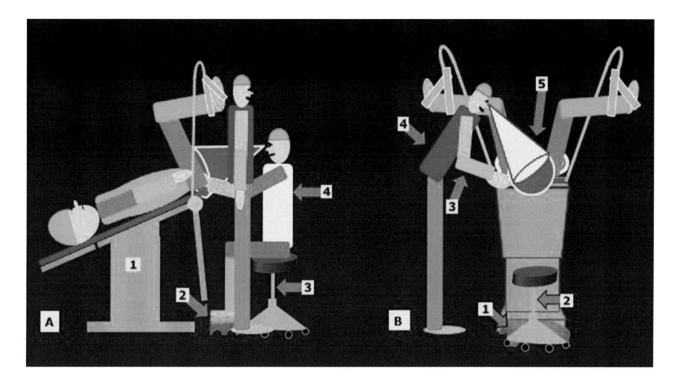

(A) Lateral view illustrating adjustments made to optimize tall surgical assistant's **(SA)** functioning.

- o **(1)** table base is raised to allow ergonomic positioning for the **SA**.
- o **(2)** positions footstool(s) to allow ergonomic positioning of the seated primary surgeon **(PS)**. Enough footstools need to be used to allow the **PS's** thigh to be parallel to the floor or the **PS** will develop cramps in the thigh caused by pressure from the edge of the sitting stool on muscles in the posterior thigh.
- o **(3)** the sitting stool is elevated to allow ergonomic positioning of the seated **PS**.
- o **(4)** illustrates ergonomic positioning for the **PS's** back and eyes, creating an optimal field of view for the **PS**.

(B) illustrates how the changes improve the ergonomic positioning for the surgical assistant.

- o **(1)** shows the footstool(s) that allow the **PS** to maintain an ergonomic seated position.
- o **(2)** shows the elevated height of the **PS's** sitting stool.
- o **(3)** shows ergonomic position of the **SA's** arms (i.e., Relaxed slight bend at the elbow with hands positioned to easily assist the **PS**). If the **SA** has to have the arms fully extended, the deltoid and pectoral muscles are under constant tension, leading to muscle fatigue for the **SA**.
- o **(4)** illustrates the **SA's** relaxed back position which minimizes muscle tension and fatigue.
- o **(5)** illustrates the fact that the **SA** field of view is the same as the **PS** field of view. This results in improved efficiency for the **PS** and **SA**.

Pressure-Induced Complications

Supine Position Pressure Points

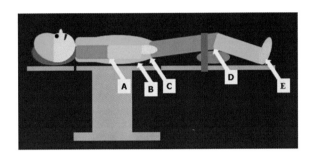

Patients in the supine position are at risk for position-related injuries due to sustained pressure from normal body weight. The anesthetized patient does not get signals from muscles to the brain to move and protect the body from injury.

- **(A)** The ulnar nerve is close to the surface and needs additional padding to prevent injury.
- **(B)** In thin patients, the sacrum is at risk for injury and needs additional padding for prolonged procedures.
- **(C)** The coccyx also needs additional padding in thin patients.
- **(D)** The legs require slight flexion using pillows under the knee to reduce strain on the lumbar spine.
- **(E)** The heel is at risk for pressure ulcers and requires additional padding for protection.

Lithotomy Trendelenburg— Candy CaneStirrups Lateral View Pressure Points

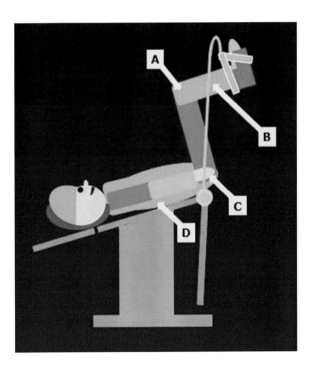

The lithotomy position is commonly used in gynecologic, urologic, and colorectal procedures. Nerve and pressure injuries may be related to positioning problems when Candy Cane Supports are used.

- **(A)** is the location of the lateral peroneal nerve. It has minimal soft tissue protection and is easily injured when the assistant leans against the leg, trapping the peroneal nerve against the Candy Cane post.
- **(B)** shows the area where the lateral peroneal nerve can be pushed into the Candy Cane pole. This happens when the assistant surgeon leans against the leg during the procedure.
- **(C)** illustrates the hand between the hip and the lower pole of the Candy Cane stirrup. The hand is at risk for a pressure or crush injury at this point. A foam pad around the hand will prevent this type of injury.
- **(D)** The ulnar and radial nerves are at risk for pressure injury when the arms are tucked. The elbow and arm need to be protected by foam padding before tucking the arm.

Lithotomy Supine— Candy Cane Stirrups Perineal View Pressure Points

The perineal view of the patient in lithotomy position with candy cane leg supports is illustrated at the left. **Key points to consider include the following:**

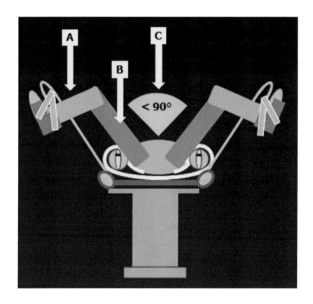

- **(A)** Knee and calf need to be away from contact with Candy Cane stirrup support pole to avoid peroneal nerve injury.
- **(B)** Medial aspect of thigh at risk for pressure injury to saphenous nerve if surgical assistant leans against thigh for prolonged time during surgical procedure.
- **(C)** Thighs abducted at no more than a ninety-degree angle due to inadvertent injury to hip joint or stretch injury to obturator nerve if greater angle occurs.

Lithotomy—Trendelenburg—Partial Flexion with Allen Stirrups Pressure Points

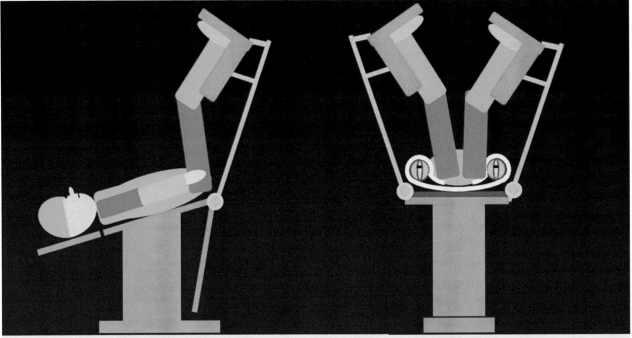

Trendelenburg Lateral View   Trendelenburg Perineal View

The above figure illustrates a lateral and perineal view of the patient in lithotomy position with Allen Stirrups. The table is in Trendelenburg at a **twenty to thirty** degree angle. The legs of the patient are elevated at **seventy to eighty** degrees from the floor. This allows the surgeon and assistant to position themselves close to the surgical field. The legs are partially flexed at the knee in stirrups to relax tension on the nerves and improve blood flow return from the extremity to the heart.

The Allen Stirrups are designed to avoid pressure-related injuries to the heel, ankle, and peroneal nerve area. ***However*, the rotation of the leg about the hip and knee increases the risks of torque injury to the ligament and joint surfaces at these locations.** These joint injuries are also considered pressure-related complications.

Scalp Pressure Point Injury

Nearly all patients having a surgical procedure in the OR will have an anesthesiologist or nurse anesthetist caring for their airway. Most often, the primary surgeon delegates care of the head to anesthesia personnel. **Yet Pressure-Induced Scalp Problems will not come back to the anesthesia personnel. They will come back to the surgeon!**

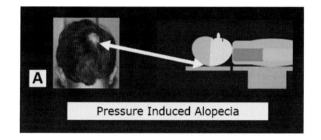
Pressure Induced Alopecia

- **(A) Pressure-Induced Alopecia**
  - ○ Prolonged pressure on the back of head may result in alopecia.
  - ○ Prolonged pressure may reduce blood supply to delicate hair follicles, causing subsequent failure to grow.
  - ○ The anesthesia provider is responsible for maintaining the head in a neutral position to protect the neck and scalp.

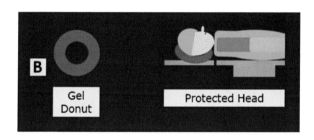
Gel Donut · Protected Head

- **(B) Protect Scalp Blood Supply**
  - ○ Use of a gel doughnut protects the occiput by decreasing pressure on the scalp and preserving blood flow to the hair follicles.

Nerve Injuries Associated with Common Positioning Errors

Prolonged surgery (>two hours) **and external compression or stretching are the most common cause of pressure-induced nerve injury.** While ulnar nerve, brachial plexus, and lumbosacral nerve injuries are the most frequently reported nerve injuries in that order, the American Society of Anesthesiologists closed claims database revealed that these injuries occurred despite documented standard of care positioning, padding, and evaluation in 63 percent of patients with perioperative neuropathies. **This information emphasizes the need to document use of positioning protocol tools used during the surgical procedure as a risk management tool.**

Upper Extremity Nerves

Brachial plexus nerve injury

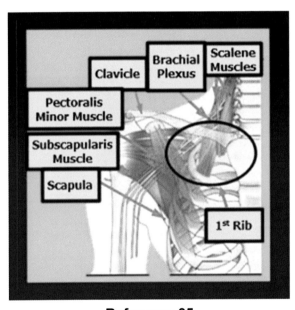

Reference 35

- **Brachial plexus injuries are the second most common peripheral nerve injury due to improper positioning of patients during surgery.**
- The brachial plexus is a network of nerves extending from the spinal cord through the neck and into the armpit, controlling sensation and muscle function in the upper extremity.
- **The key to diagnosing post-op pressure-induced brachial plexus nerve injuries is being aware of the soft signs of sensory and/or muscle action loss of the five major nerves that make up the Brachial Plexus.**
- Brachial plexus nerve injuries are caused by stretching or compressing the nerve plexus **between the clavicle and the first rib.**

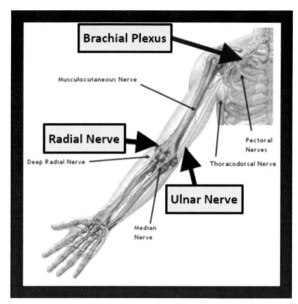

- The illustration at the left reveals the major nerve anatomic relationships in the upper extremity.

- **The most common nerves associated with positioning pressure-induced neuropathies are highlighted.**

Reference 36

How Does Brachial Plexus Nerve Injury Occur?

Brachial Plexus Injury from Arm Board > Ninety Degrees Abduction

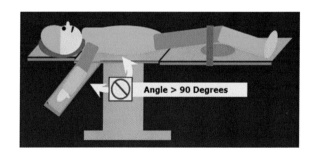

- Abduction of the arm should be limited to less than ninety degrees from the chest. If angle of abduction is greater than ninety degrees, stretch injuries to the multiple nerves may occur.

Brachial Plexus Injury from Neck Turned Away from Arm on Arm Board

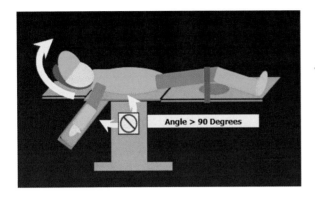

- Brachial plexus injuries can also occur when the neck is turned away **(arrow at head)** from the arm on the arm board. This is another stretch injury to the nerves.

Brachial Plexus Injury Associated with Inappropriate Tucking of Arm

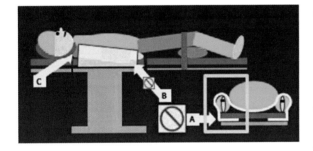

- **(A)** Lift sheet tucking arm between mattress and OR table. The sheet between the mattress and the table is easily dislodged by any lateral movement/pressure on the arm, allowing the arm to fall off the OR table.
- **(B)** Hand and wrist are loosely restrained and may easily flop off of the mattress.
- **(C)** Shoulder pulled down by lift sheet between mattress and OR table stretching brachial plexus nerves when the arm falls off the table.

Brachial Plexus Injury When Arm Falls Off Table

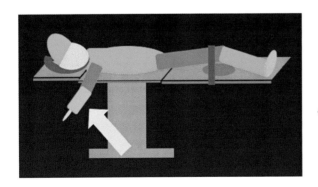

- Arm falling off OR table increases stretch on brachial plexus nerves.

Ulnar Nerve Injury

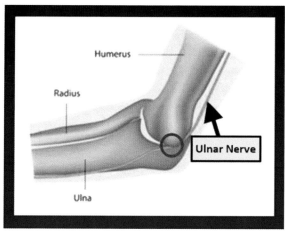

Ref 37

- **The most common nerve injury in the anesthetized patient is the ulnar nerve.**
- The etiology of this injury is reported to be compression or stretching of the nerve associated with a prolonged surgical procedure.
- Men's bones are normally larger than women's bones and are associated with a narrower groove for the ulnar nerve to pass through. This anatomic variant creates a higher risk for ulnar nerve impingement at the elbow joint.
- The drawing at the left illustrates the area of the ulnar nerve most vulnerable to position-related injury during surgery.

Arm Position on Arm Board to Prevent Ulnar Nerve Injury

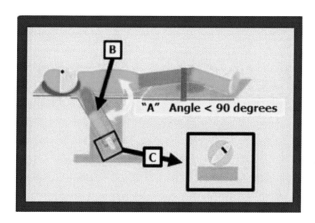

- Correct positioning of the arm on the arm board.
  - o **(A)** Arm is less than ninety degrees to the thorax.
  - o **(B)** Forearm is slightly flexed (twenty degrees) from straight line.
  - o **(C)** Palm is rotated twenty to thirty degrees from flat on the arm board.
- This position relaxes the tension on the ulnar nerve, as it crosses the elbow and protects the nerve in the natural groove above the olecranon.

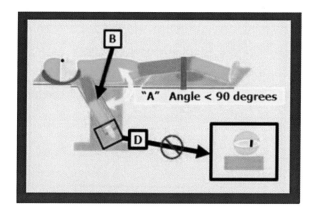

- Incorrect positioning of the arm on the arm board.
  - o **(A)** Arm is less than ninety degrees to the thorax.
  - o **(B)** Forearm is slightly flexed (twenty degrees) from straight line.
  - o **(D)** *Palm is flat on the arm board, exposing the ulnar nerve to increased pressure at the elbow.*
  - o If the patient were awake, this position causes pain. The patient would automatically rotate the hand to relieve pain if awake.

Surgical Assistant Creating Ulnar Nerve Pressure-Induced Injury

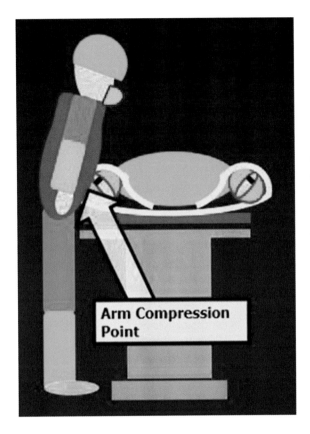

Arm Compression Point

- Pressure injuries (leaning on the patient).
- The surgical assistant in this illustration is placing pressure against the arm, compressing the ulnar nerve at the elbow joint.
- The risk of this injury occurring increases with the number of assistants trying to position themselves to see the surgical field.

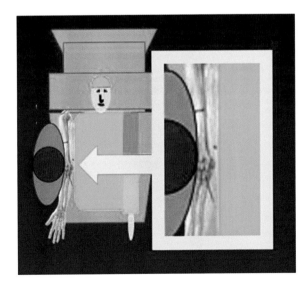

- Overhead view shows the assistant surgeon leaning against the tucked arm at the level of the elbow. *The anatomic inset reveals the arm in the palm-up position so the ulnar nerve at the elbow can be seen.* The tucked arm would have the ulnar nerve adjacent to the bone joint, and pressure against the arm would compress the ulnar nerve **(arrow)**, resulting in compromised blood flow to the nerve.

Ulnar Nerve Injury Symptoms

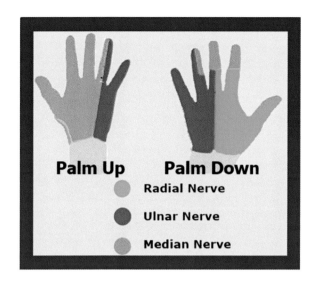

• Loss of sensation of lateral portion of ring finger and sensation of little finger

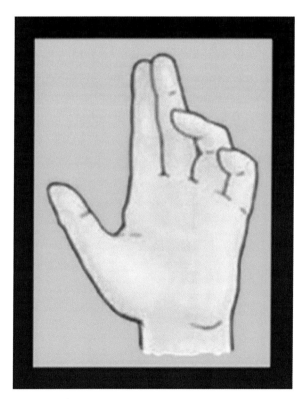

• Inability to abduct or oppose the fifth finger
• Weakness of grasp with fourth and fifth fingers
• Pain in the medial forearm

Radial Nerve

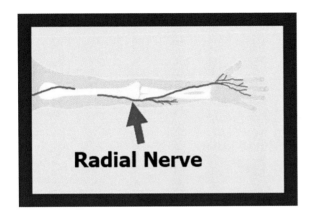

Radial Nerve

- The radial nerve crosses under the humerus bone and over the lateral epicondyle on its way to the medial aspect of the wrist.

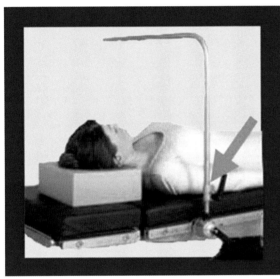

Ref 38

- When anesthesia uses a screen attached **(arrow)** to the side rails of the OR table, it can compress the soft tissue of the arm, resulting in a pressure injury to the radial nerve.

Radial Nerve Injury Symptoms

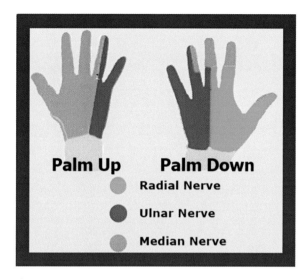

- Loss of sensation on back of thumb and index finger

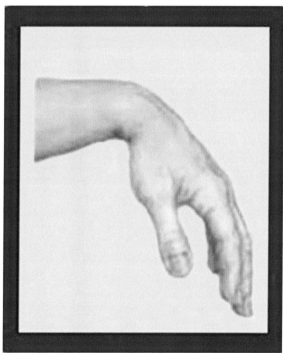

- Inability to extend fingers
- Inability to extend wrist (wrist-drop)
- Pain in the medial forearm

Axillary Nerve Injury Symptoms

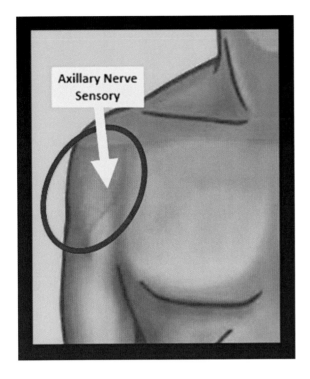

- Numbness and tingling occur in the shoulder area.
- Decreased sensation to the lateral shoulder.
- Inability to abduct the arm.
- Impaired deltoid muscle function, resulting in difficulty lifting arm above the head.

Musculocutaneous Nerve Injury Symptoms

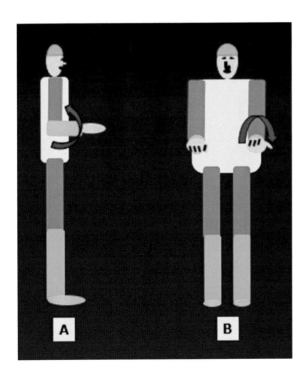

- Sensory loss to the lateral portion of the forearm
- **(A)**
  - Inability to flex forearm
  - Inability to flex biceps
- **(B)**
  - Unable to rotate forearm to have palm face up

Lower Extremity Nerve Injuries Associated with Positioning Errors

Sciatic Nerve

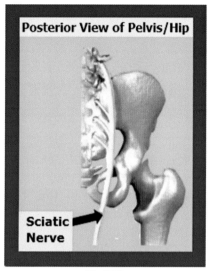

Ref 39

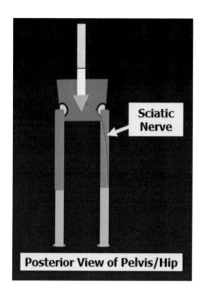

- The Sciatic Nerve is a combination of the L4, L5, S1, S2, and S3 spinal nerve branches.
- It provides both motor and sensory functions to the lower extremity.
- It divides into two main branches behind the knee **(The Tibial Nerve and the Common Peroneal Nerve).**

- **The Sciatic Nerve is easily injured by excessive flexion of the thigh toward the abdomen when positioned in the lithotomy position for surgery.** Since the patient is asleep, the patient cannot adjust painful leg positions in the lithotomy position to relieve pain.

- Lying in the supine position maintains normal tension on the Sciatic Nerve.

- A neutral lithotomy position will also maintain normal tension on the Sciatic Nerve.

- **Symptoms of Sciatic Nerve injury include the following:**
  - Pain is one-sided in the hip or buttocks.
  - Pain may be constant.
  - Pain gets worse with sitting.
  - Pain radiates down the leg and increases when trying to stand.

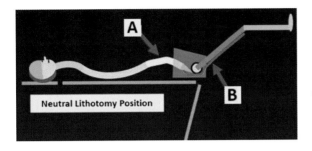

The stirrups (candy cane or Allen) are not illustrated in this diagram to allow clear demonstration of the anatomic position of the nerves, spine, legs, and pelvis.

- In the neutral lithotomy position, the Sciatic Nerve has no compression on the soft tissue surrounding it.
- **(A)** The Lumbar-Sacral lordotic curve remains normal.
- **(B)** No increased stretching of the Sciatic Nerve as it courses through the soft tissue.

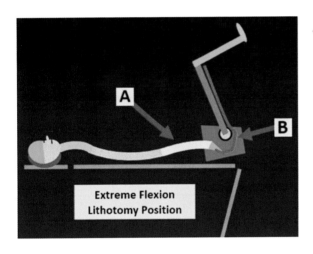

The stirrups (candy cane or Allen) are not illustrated in this diagram to allow clear demonstration of the anatomic position of the nerves, spine, legs, and pelvis.

- When the patient is positioned in extreme flexion (>one hundred degrees from the supine plane),

  (A) the lordotic curve of the spine flattens and can cause significant postoperative pain and

  (B) the Sciatic Nerve is stretched and compressed against the pelvic bony structures, resulting in compromised sensory and motor function in the distribution of the nerve.

- **The impact of this problem is increased if a member of the surgical team leans against the leg while attempting to assist the surgeon.**

Femoral Nerve

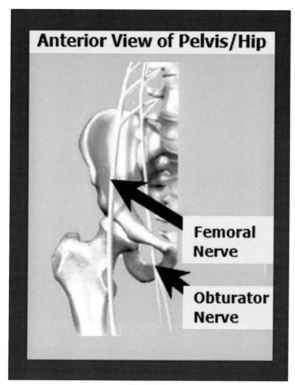

Anterior View of Pelvis/Hip

Femoral Nerve

Obturator Nerve

Ref 40

Femoral Nerve Function

The Femoral Nerve provides both motor and sensory control to the lower extremity. Motor control involves the major hip flexor muscles and knee extension muscles. The anterior branch provides sensory function to the thigh. The posterior branch becomes the Saphenous Nerve, providing sensory function to a portion of the lower leg and foot.

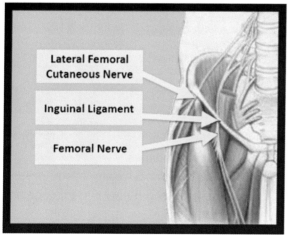

Lateral Femoral Cutaneous Nerve

Inguinal Ligament

Femoral Nerve

Ref 41

- Both the Femoral Nerve and Lateral Femoral Cutaneous Nerve enter the lower extremity by passing under the inguinal ligament.
- Extreme flexion and abduction of the thighs may place pressure on these nerves, impacting their function.
- Symptoms may include
  - numbness usually in anterior lateral aspect of the thigh,
  - difficulty extending the knee due to quadriceps weakness,
  - feeling like your knee is going to buckle on you.

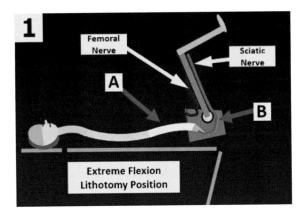

Figure 1

- **(A)** Flattening of Lumbar Spine curve, resulting in low back pain postoperatively.
- **(B)** Stretching of Sciatic Nerve due to excessive flexion of thigh.

Figure 2

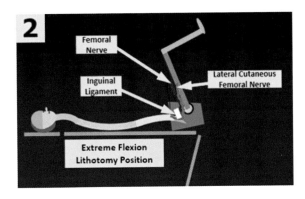

- Femoral Nerve and Lateral Cutaneous Femoral Nerve are crimped when the thighs are flexed excessively in the lithotomy position.
- Patients may have sensory-loss symptoms in the distribution of either or both nerves postoperatively when extreme flexion of the legs occurs while using the lithotomy position for surgery.

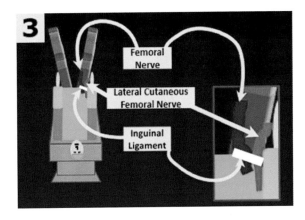

Figure 3

- Overhead view of the patient in extreme flexion using the lithotomy position.
- Note how the Inguinal Ligament compresses the nerves passing below it in this position.

Obturator Nerve

The Obturator Nerve provides motor stimulus to the adductor muscles of the lower limb and sensory function to the medial aspect of the thigh.

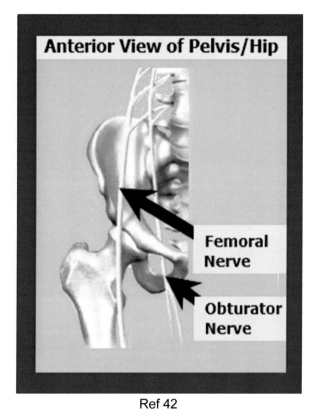

Ref 42

- The Obturator Nerve is injured as it exits the obturator foramen when the thigh is flexed excessively. The injury is a stretch injury of the nerve.

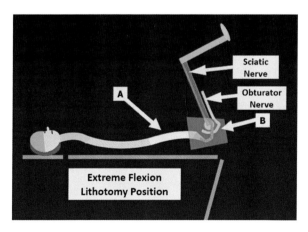

- Extreme flexion of the leg onto the abdomen or extreme abduction of the leg can lead to stretch injuries of the Obturator Nerve and Sciatic Nerve.
- **(A)** Excessive flexion of the legs flattens the lumbar spine and may result in postoperative low back pain.
- **(B)** As the pelvis is lifted off the OR table, the Obturator and Sciatic Nerves are placed on stretch.

Perineal View of Obturator and Sciatic Nerves

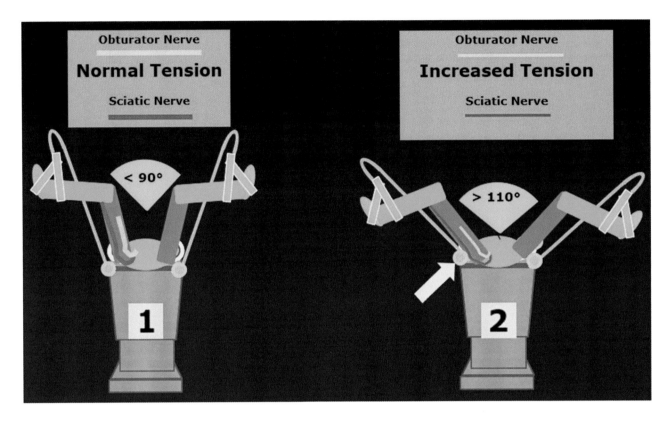

- Figure 1 shows a neutral lithotomy position using Candy Cane stirrups. The knees are slightly flexed, and the thighs are abducted at less than ninety degrees to protect the hip joints.
- This position maintains normal tension on the Obturator and Sciatic Nerves.
- The picture does not show protective padding at points of pressure to enable visualization of body parts to OR table support structures.

- Figure 2 shows the Candy Cane stirrups abducted at an angle greater than 110°. The wide-open angle creates torque on the hip joint with potential postoperative hip pain (arrow).
- The increased extension of the legs stretches and decreases the diameter of the Obturator and Sciatic Nerves. The associated reduced blood flow may cause postoperative nerve dysfunction.
- The picture does not show protective padding at points of pressure to enable visualization of body parts to OR table support structures.

Common Peroneal Nerve Injury

The **Common Peroneal Nerve** is the smaller and terminal branch of the **Sciatic Nerve**. It courses along the upper lateral side of the popliteal fossa, deep to the biceps-femoris muscle and its tendon until it gets to the posterior part of the head of the fibula.

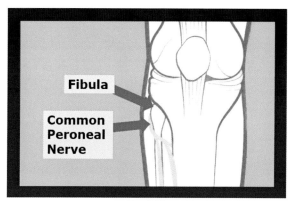

Ref 43

- Injury to the Peroneal Nerve is common because of its exposure on the lateral aspect of the knee.
- The injury occurs when patients have their legs elevated in the lithotomy position and the poorly protected nerve is compressed against the stirrup pole for Candy Cane stirrups or the unpadded edge of the Allen Stirrup supportive boot.
- Injury is easily prevented by properly positioning the leg away from the stirrup pole or adequately padding the top of the Allen Stirrup boot.

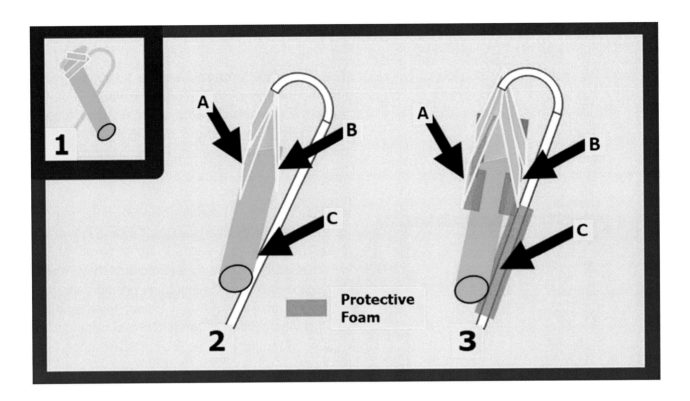

1. **Inset** showing leg and foot in a Candy Cane stirrup supported by straps around the foot and ankle.
2. View is rotated, showing the foot and ankle unprotected in the straps and the leg contacting the pole of the Candy Cane Stirrup.

   (A) The edge of the Candy Cane strap on the medial aspect of the leg can put pressure on the Tibial Nerve, resulting in postoperative nerve compression symptoms.

   (B) The edge of the Candy Cane strap on the lateral aspect of the leg can put pressure on the Superficial Peroneal Nerve, resulting in postoperative nerve compression symptoms.

   (C) The leg is in contact with the Candy Cane Pole, placing pressure on the Peroneal Nerve and resulting in postoperative nerve compression symptoms.

3. The foot and ankle are protected by a foam boot between the foot and the straps supporting the leg in the Candy Cane stirrup. The knee and upper portion of the leg are protected by using foam wrapped about the Candy Cane stirrup pole.

   (A) The Tibial Nerve is separated from the strap by the foam boot.
   (B) The Superficial Peroneal Nerve is protected by the foam boot.
   (C) Pressure on the Peroneal Nerve is minimized by covering the Candy Cane Stirrup pole with foam.

Random Pearls for Rare Position Problems

Ischemic Optic Neuropathy (ION)

- Ophthalmic injuries occur between 0.1 percent and 1.0 percent of surgical cases
- ION is a rare but potentially catastrophic complication associated with steep Trendelenburg surgical positioning and prolonged surgical times.
- Symptoms include blurred or lost vision postoperatively.
- The etiology of ION is felt to be related to increased intraocular pressure.
- Studies have demonstrated intraocular pressure is increased significantly with steep Trendelenburg position and prolonged surgery.

Compartment Syndrome

- Acute compartment syndrome is a rare but serious complication related to surgical positioning.
- It occurs in patients who have had long surgical procedures usually involving the lithotomy position.
- Compartment syndrome of the lower leg is associated with hypoperfusion of the lower leg tissues and pressure on the tissues related to the type of support of the lower extremity in the lithotomy position.
- The associated tissue ischemia creates leakage of fluid into closed muscle compartments, resulting in more ischemia.
- Fasciotomy is required to relieve increased pressure.
- If not recognized early and treated aggressively, sepsis, loss of the limb, or even death may occur.
- Primary signs and symptoms include
  - pain disproportionate to physical findings;
  - pain not responsive to analgesics, including parenteral opiates;
  - tense, hard compartment tissues;
  - lost pulses.
- Diagnosis should be considered for any patient with a procedure lasting three hours or more.
- Upper extremity compartment syndrome may be associated with malfunctioning of blood pressure cuffs or excessive pressure from positioning restraints.

Epilogue

While society normally associates patient surgical outcome with the surgeon performing the surgery, the surgical outcome for patients is actually the result of how well the surgical team performs the nonsurgical functions. The pearls discussed in this primer are non-surgical actions performed by surgical team members and known to impact surgical outcome. The actions discussed by the authors were distilled from thousands of hours spent by the authors in the OR during their active surgical careers. Nonsurgical issues were separated from issues involving specific surgical techniques. **Simple tasks not performed appropriately can lead to poor patient outcomes despite appropriate performance of the primary surgical procedure.** Some of the rare perioperative cases discussed in this primer were identified from cases presented to the authors to review because of bad patient outcomes following common surgical procedures.

The authors value your comments regarding the information presented in this primer and can be reached at GMTigerBooksLLC@gmail.com

Appendix A

Download PDF copy of form below at www.gmtigerbooksllc.net

Patient Name: _____ Date of Surgery: _____

Name of Surgery Facility: _____ Primary Procedure: _____ Surgeon: _____

ELPO Pressure Injury Risk Assessment Scale Date of Assessment: _____

Item \ Score	5	4	3	2	1	Value
Surgical Position	• Lithotomy	• Prone	• Trendelenburg	• Lateral	• Supine	
Surgery Duration	• Over 6 hr.	• More than 4 hr. Up to 6 hr.	• More than 2 hr. Up to 4 hr.	• More than 1 hr. Up to 2 hr.	• Less than 1 hr.	
Anesthesia Type	• General + Regional	• General	• Regional	• Sedation	• Local	
Support Surface: • OR Table • Limbs	• Thin pad • Thin or no pad	• Foam pad • Sheets or towels	• Foam pad • Foam pad	• Foam Pad • Viscoelastic pad	• Viscoelastic pad • Viscoelastic pad	
Limb Position	• Knees raised >90° • Lower limbs open >90° • Upper limbs open >90°	• Knees raised >90° • Lower limbs open >90°	• Knees raised <90° • Lower limbs open <90° • Neck without sternal alignment	• Upper limbs open <90°	• Anatomic position • Arms tucked palm to hip	
Comorbidities	History of: • Pressure ulcer • Neuropathy • Deep venous thrombosis	• Obesity (BMI > 35) • Malnutrition (BMI < 18.5)	• Diabetes Mellitus	• Vascular disease	• No comorbidities	
Patient age	• >80 years	• 70 to 79 years	• 60 to 69 years	• 40 to 59 years	• 18 to 39 years	
					Total Score:	

Total score > 20 at increased risk for pressure induced injury.

Special equipment required in OR.

1.	4.
2.	5.
3.	6.
7.	
8.	
9.	

References:

Reference #	Reference
1	*Houston Chronicle.* **May 13, 2000.**
2	*Houston Chronicle.* **May 13, 2000.**
3	Lopes, C. M. de M., V. J. Haas, R. A. S. Dantas, C.G. de Oliveira, and C. M. Galvao. 2016. "Assessment Scale of Risk for Surgical Positioning Injuries". *Revista Latino Americana de Enfermagem*, 24, e2704. Retrieved from http://doi.org/10.1590/1518-8345.0644.2704.
4	https://www.ansell.com/ca/en/products/sandel-ergo-step-stool
5	https://www.wayfair.com/furniture/pdp/inbox-zero-round-rolling-pu-leather-height-adjustable-lab-stool-w003193010.html?piid=2094739360
6	https://www.alimed.com/single-post-mayo-stand.html?pid=164825
7	https://www.graylinemedical.com/products/bovie-medical-corporation-bovie-ids-generators-electrosurgical-generator-ids-200-ids210?variant=31849512337465
8	https://www.cardinalhealth.com/en/product-solutions/medical/compression/a-v-impulse-foot-compression-system.html
9	https://www.cardinalhealth.com/en/product-solutions/medical/compression/kendall-scd-compression-system.html
10	https://www.3m.com/3M/en_US/company-us/all-3m-products/~/All-3M-Products/Health-Care/Medical/Surgical-Safety-Solutions/Patient-Warming-Blankets/?N=5002385+7570653+8707795+8707798+8711017+8711100+8711119+3294857497&rt=r3
11	https://www.cardinalhealth.com/en/product-solutions/medical/infection-control/fluid-management/medi-vac-suction-canisters.html
12	https://www.medtronic.com/covidien/en-us/products/smoke-evacuation/rapidvac-smoke-evacuator-system.html
13	https://www.hillrom.com/en/products/patient-transfer-boards/
14	https://hovermatt.com/products/hovermatt-air-transfer-system/
15	https://www.steris.com/healthcare/products/surgical-lights-and-examination-lights/surgical-lights/harmonyair-e-series-surgical-lighting-system
16	https://www.jnjmedicaldevices.com/en-US/product/ethicon-gen11-generator

Reference #	Reference
17	https://www.conmed.com/en/products/laparoscopic-robotic-and-open-surgery/energy/argon-beam-technology/helixar-electrosurgical-generator-with-argon-beam-coagulation-abc
18	https://lumenis.com/medical/co2-products/#ultrapulse-family
19	https://lumenis.com/medical/holmium-products/#versapulse-family
20	https://www.siemens-healthineers.com/en-us/surgical-c-arms-and-navigation/mobile-c-arms/cios-alpha-cmos
21	https://www.gehealthcare.com/products/ultrasound/logiq
22	https://www.medtronic.com/us-en/healthcare-professionals/products/cardiovascular/blood-management-diagnostics/autolog-autotransfusion-system.html
23	https://www.sklarcorp.com/retractors/abdominal-retractors
24	https://www.ebay.com/sch/i.html?_from=R40&_trksid=p2380057.m570.l1313&_nkw=O%27Connor-O%27Sullivan+Retractor&_sacat=0
25	https://www.ebay.com/sch/i.html?_from=R40&_trksid=p2380057.m570.l1313&_nkw=Turner+Warwick+retractor&_sacat=0
26	https://www.surgicalholdings.co.uk/bookwalter-retractor.html
27	https://www.appliedmedical.com/Products/Alexis/OWoundProtectorRetractor
28	https://www.coopersurgical.com/medical-devices/surgical/?min=0&max=0&mn=&vn=&tp=&prop=1346&filters=product-brand%5B126%5D
29	https://www.surgicalspecialties.com/suture-wound-closure-brands/quill-barbed-sutures/
30	https://www.jnjmedicaldevices.com/en-US/search-hcp?search_api_fulltext=stratafix
31	https://www.3m.com/3M/en_US/company-us/all-3m-products/~/d/hcbgdgm20045/
32	https://www.hillrom.com/en/products/stirrups/

Reference #	Reference
33	Souki, F. G., Y.F. Rodriguez-Blanco, S.R. Polu, et al. "Survey of Anesthesiologists' Practices Related to Steep Trendelenburg Positioning in the USA." *BMC Anesthesiol* **18**, 117 (2018).
34	https://openi.nlm.nih.gov/detailedresult?img=PMC3428177_PAMJ-12-57-g001&query=periorbital%20edema&it=xg&req=4&npos=40
35	https://bioanadrasis.com/%CE%B1%CF%85%CF%87%CE%B5%CE%BD%CE%B9%CE%BA%CF%8C-%CE%BF%CE%B9-101-%CE%B1%CE%B9%CF%84%CE%AF%CE%B5%CF%82-%CF%80%CE%BF%CF%85-%CF%84%CE%BF-%CF%80-%CF%81%CE%BF%CE%BA%CE%B1%CE%BB%CE%BF%CF%8D%CE%BD/brachial-plexus-4-3/
36	https://www.pinterest.com/pin/780178335420074505
37	https://premierneurologycenter.com/conditions-treatment/ulnar-neuropathy/
38	https://www.schuremed.com/anesthesia-screen.html
39	https://miamineurosciencecenter.com/en/conditions/sciatica/
40	https://www.lecturio.com/concepts/hip-joint/
41	https://www.aafp.org/afp/2000/0401/p2109.html
42	https://www.lecturio.com/concepts/hip-joint/
43	https://www.kneeguru.co.uk/KNEEnotes/knee-dictionary/common-peroneal-nerve

Illustration Credit

All tables, diagrams, and illustrations not specifically referenced in the bibliography were designed and created for this primer by Carl F. Giesler.

Printed in the United States
by Baker & Taylor Publisher Services